Moments of Being

Moments of Being

The Random Recollections of
Raymond Greene

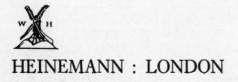

HEINEMANN : LONDON

William Heinemann Ltd
15 Queen St, Mayfair, London W1X 8BE

LONDON MELBOURNE TORONTO
JOHANNESBURG AUCKLAND

First published in 1974
Copyright © Raymond Greene 1974
Reprinted 1974

SBN 434 305731

Printed in Great Britain by
Redwood Burn Limited
Trowbridge and Esher

Contents

Illustrations

Acknowledgements

The author is indebted to the following for permission to reproduce illustrations: *The Daily Telegraph* for that of Georg Scheurrer; The Radio Times Hulton Picture Library for The Beast 666; Mr J. Roderick Cameron and the Royal College of Surgeons Edinburgh for Joseph Ryland Whitaker and his class; The Royal Geographical Society for the Everest Expedition in Sikkim and Frank Smythe and Eric Shipton.

Preface

I want, dear reader, to be a camera (to borrow a phrase from my cousin Christopher Isherwood) and not a mirror. You, looking over my shoulder into a mirror held before my face could hardly be interested unless I were a person of supreme importance to you – Winston Churchill perhaps, or someone you have loved. The face in the mirror of an ordinary physician would be very boring. But if you had the privilege of sharing with him the view-finder of his camera, it would not matter how boring he himself might be – you would share with him the funny or interesting or exciting things that he had seen. That is my object and I can assure the reader who shares my view-finder that I will switch the camera as seldom as possible towards my person, and that no place or person or incident in this narrative is entirely imaginary.

I have omitted my childhood, which was happy and free from incident. I saw nothing horrible in the woodshed, perhaps because we had no woodshed. My affection for the rocking horse that I shared with my five brothers and sisters was purely platonic.

R.G.

1 Lead In

People climb mountains for a lot of different reasons: because it is a game of skill, or because they like lovely country or hard exercise in the fresh air, or because they want to appear rather tough to themselves or other people, and sometimes for scientific reasons, because they are botanists or geologists or physiologists. But for quite a lot of climbers the most powerful reason – if you call it a reason – is an itch to get to the top of a thing and see what's on the other side. It doesn't matter a lot whether the thing is a road dipping over the skyline of a Sussex hill or the waste of ice and rock on a Himalayan mountainside; but on a mountainside you have all the other reasons for climbing coming in too. It was fun at twelve years old to get to the top of Catbells, a little green mountain in Cumberland, but it was more exciting to get to the Himalaya long afterwards.

My father loved mountains and walking in them, but he was never a climber in the sense of frequenting places where a rope round the waist was a necessity. Perhaps he had in his youth the itch to climb; he certainly encouraged the itch in his children. Only Molly, my elder sister, shared it with me. With our father, sometimes our Aunt Nora, sometimes friends of his with boys that were coaching for higher examinations, we went every summer to the English Lake District, staying usually at Stool End, the home of the Martindales, at the head of Great Langdale where the valley splits into Oxendale, leading up to Bowfell, and Mickleden, leading to Rossett Ghyll and the Stake Pass to Borrowdale. Scenically it is unchanged today. The 'pension' in those days was five shillings a head. That has changed. Sometimes we stayed at Wall End, a mile down the valley, sometimes at Middle Fell, the home of Dick Wilson in Wasdale. We walked what seem to me now immense distances over the fells. There is not a peak in the central fells we did not climb. My father was indefatigable and we were very young. My first mountain, when I was twelve years old, was Catbells, just qualifying for the title of mountain at 1,481 feet, the home of Mrs Tiggy-Winkle, lying above Little-town where Sally Henny-penny 'went bare foot, bare foot'.

I was sixteen years old when Ashley Abrahams, the great pioneer of English rock-climbing, came to lecture at Berkhamsted. The boys crowded round him afterwards and I told him that I had walked his native fells for four years. 'Come and see me,' he said, 'next time. I will find you someone who will teach you real climbing.' In the next year I took him at his word and went to see him at his photographer's shop in Keswick. He introduced me to a lone climber called Binns who took me up the Napes Needle. The obsession was born.

The next year Abrahams introduced me to Weeks, with whom I did the Needle again and other climbs of moderate difficulty. I fell in with Holland and Speaker, great rock climbers in their day. I especially remember the day when the three of us polished off in one day all the climbs then known on the Napes. We did not stop for lunch and it was only as I ran rejoicing back to Langdale that I knew I was hungry.

In 1920 Charles Holland, my sister Molly and I had a wonderful day on Pillar Rock. We descended by the New West climb. I led down, Molly between us, Holland, as befitting the most experienced climber, in the rear. We came to a place where we climbed down a vertical 'chimney', and struck out horizontally on a traverse before descending vertically again. I took up my stance at the end of the traverse, but, being inexperienced, did not belay myself and merely took in the rope as Molly climbed across to me. I assumed that Holland would be, as he should have been, protecting her with her rope above. Suddenly she fell, and, instead of being supported by Holland, she plunged downwards. The rope ran through my hands until, about fifty feet below, she struck a grass ledge, and was

2

momentarily halted before bouncing off again. At this moment I twisted her rope round my forearm and stopped her. The rope between her and Holland had almost run out and he, against all the rules, was himself climbing down the chimney. Had I not stopped her when I did, he would have been pulled off. I could not have held them both and all three of us would have been killed. In fact, Molly had no injury except minor cuts and bruises, and I only a flayed hand.

My left arm was in a sling when I arrived for my first term at Pembroke, and the news that I had had a climbing accident reached the ears of Herbert Carr, also at Pembroke. He was my senior by several years, having served in the Kaiser's war. He was the architect of my mountain career. Together with Jack Wolfenden and others we reformed the Oxford University Mountaineering Club. We usually had a 'meet' in Wales in January, in Cumberland at Easter and in the Swiss Alps in summer. There was then no Cambridge mountaineering club and we always invited climbers from 'the other place' to join us. Once I had a 'return match' in Cambridge, the most terrifying weekend of my life. We did all the standard climbs on the colleges and finally Eliot Wallis, Gilbert Adair and I attempted King's Chapel. We failed high up at an overhang, but a fortnight later I had a card from the other two. They had succeeded. By stretching out the left arm, they had succeeded in holding a lightning conductor between finger and thumb, thus keeping their balance as they surmounted the drip course that had defeated us.

2 German Adventures

Because of my many other activities I was broke in 1923, and my third alpine season, by which I hoped to achieve membership of the Alpine Club, looked beyond my means. At this point a letter arrived from Mrs Hopkins, the former matron at my old house at school. A friend of hers, Irish by birth, the widow of a German officer, was earning her living as governess to a small boy in Bavaria, the only child of a German cavalry captain killed in the war and his American wife. He was only eight years old, but, in a purely feminine household, had become unmanageable. The salary seemed to me then enormous, and I accepted. With this wealth so imminent I spent three weeks with the Oxford Mountaineering Club in Switzerland, three cloudless weeks in which we ascended twenty-one peaks and passes. Then, tearing myself away, I took the train to Garmisch.

For three months more of cloudless blue I lived in the Villa Lützenkirchen with Hanno, with whom I was immediately on the most friendly terms, and his mother Louise Mayer, still in deep mourning for her husband.

The mark had slumped without my knowledge during my journey from Switzerland. The first indication of this was in a large hotel in Munich where I gave a handful of small Swiss coins in part payment, as I thought, of my somewhat excessive bill, and received in change a supply of German money which seemed to me at the time to be wealth beyond the dreams of avarice. There were two million marks to the pound.

This was, I suppose, almost the last day on which such a transaction was possible. The days were gone when travel in Germany was a source of actual profit, and visitors passed the frontier with empty trunks to return a few days later cheerfully willing to pay an almost negligible duty on their purchases. After the first week in August 1923 prices in Germany showed a regrettable tendency to rise as the exchange sank. But they were always a little slow, and foreign money was still an advantage. Mrs Mayer's comfortable portion was invested in Holland.

There followed the August cash shortage. The inflation had hardly begun, but the prices were rising at an almost incredible pace. One morning I noticed in the village that the price of a photograph I wanted was two hundred thousand marks. Walking past a neighbouring 'beauty spot' that same afternoon, I found that the price was four hundred thousand. Scandalized that there should be such a difference in price between the village and the profiteering 'beauty spot', I returned to buy it in the village. The price had risen to eight hundred thousand marks. Naturally a week of such increment produced a shortage of cash. Sometimes it was no good having English money; the banks had no notes to give in exchange. Cash was rationed. The queue would begin to line up outside the local bank at 2.00 a.m. and there was always a free fight when the doors were opened at 10.00 a.m. Then, as likely as not, one was given enough to buy a postage stamp and no more.

A cash shortage in more normal times would not have been so serious. The people would have existed on an extended system of credit. But credit in a country where a fortune on Monday night might be worthless on Tuesday is an obvious impossibility. If you could not pay your million marks for a loaf of bread there was no putting it down to your account. The loaf would probably cost two millions tomorrow. You paid cash down or you did without. Most people did the latter. The salaried classes and the pensioners were reduced to a state of destitution. The retired army officer on a handsome pension could not live a day on his year's income. The university professor took to typing and sold his library for a song. A musician I knew sold his piano for the price of a week's lodging, but decided that life without it could not be supported.

The casual Englishman saw little of this. He saw a boundless extravagance – drinking, dancing, music – and he wrote to the English papers that the German people were rich, that they had money to throw about. But what was the good of saving money which tomorrow, even this afternoon, would be almost valueless? There were two things to do: to buy English or American money if possible, and failing this to extract from what one had the maximum of purchasing power. Money changed hands like hot potatoes; fifty years' saving would be useless in a week. 'Let us eat, drink and be merry.'

The economically inexperienced and harassed Government saw only one way out of the appalling cash shortage. They printed at an increased pace. During the three months I was in the country the mark fell from two millions to 3,000 millions. Another month saw it at twenty billions. Almost every day the design of the notes was changed until they reached a bewildering variety. I said to a shopkeeper: 'How do you know this note is not a forgery?' 'I don't know,' he said, 'but what does it matter if it is?'

It was only at the end of August that the German people lost faith in their own money. This loss was brought about largely by the introduction of the multiplicator and the nominal stabilizing of prices by the introduction of the hypothetical gold mark. Each article was priced in gold marks. One multiplied this price by a number, posted in all the banks and altered three times a day, which represented the value of the mark on the international exchange. The standard was the dollar. And so it came about that the German people paid, in fact though not in theory, in dollars. They began to collect all manner of foreign currency. Then the Government stepped in and confiscated it all and made a very handsome profit by compensating in paper marks. Where a week before a shopkeeper would give you almost anything you liked for a pound note, now he shied from it as from the plague. He had been that way before. It is hardly to be wondered at that talk in Germany during this period was entirely of money, and the state of the multiplicator. Only a few original minds occasionally managed to rise to the dizzy heights of a discussion as to how this state could be remedied.

It was such a Germany that I left in early October 1923. I returned in January 1924. During my absence the crisis of the disease had been reached and passed. The rentenmark had entered the field, prices had been completely stabilized, wages had risen almost in proportion, and the exchange had settled down comfortably at a fixed 18 billion marks to the pound, a figure rather humorous in view of the fact that the old mark had completely ceased to exist. The rentenmark, eighteen to the pound, always known as the 'mark', had put the German people on its feet as far as internal affairs were concerned. Money was beginning to lose favour as a subject of conversation. The German people were very poor, but they knew where they stood.

I returned for the third time in September 1924. The Dawes Report had been accepted by the London Conference and, a few days after my arrival, by the Reichstag. Optimism prevailed. Nationalism had once more begun to crow. Credit had been re-established on a normal basis. It was no longer necessary to spend every penny one earned without pause for thought. The casual Englishman said things were very bad. There was less gaiety in the cafés and hotels than in 1923, for your mark today would be a mark tomorrow.

In Garmisch I mixed freely with all Frau Mayer's friends. There was no atmosphere of antisemitism in Bavaria in 1923. Frau Mayer's late husband was a Jew, but this seemed not to matter. Amongst others who came to the Villa Lützenkirchen was General Karl Haushofer, a relative by marriage. I remember the clipped lawn in the sunshine, full of people against the background of the Wettersteingebirge, the loveliest bit of mountain architecture in Europe, perhaps in the world. I wanted to talk to Resi who stood, alone for once, under the mulberry tree, but Frau Bassermann wouldn't stop explaining to me how her late husband the Chancellor and the Kaiser himself had tried to prevent the war; hand in glove they had been, but the generals wouldn't listen. An angel flew across the sunshine and I heard the voice of General Haushofer who, I had been told, had commanded the German artillery at the battle of the Somme. He was talking to my employer, Mrs Mayer. 'Do you know,' he was saying, 'I didn't think I could ever like an Englishman but I like that young tutor of yours. Do you think he would like to come to my house in München?'

Dinner with the Haushofers. I didn't know then that fat old Frau Haushofer was a Jewess and I wouldn't have been interested anyway. The General said grace and without a pause, while we were regaining our chairs, said, 'You know we have Raymond with us and his German is not yet very good. We can all speak English and I suggest that this evening we should speak only English, even to each other. It will be more fun for Raymond and good for us.' Courtesy could go no further.

With Albrecht his son I formed one of those sudden temporary intimacies of the very young. We climbed together in the Wetterstein. He was an enthusiastic but not very expert mountaineer. Once on an easy pitch he fell off and I held him safely on the rope. How could I guess that twenty years later he would fall from a more difficult pitch and that the rope that time would not be round his waist? He had no hint of Jewishness in his appearance. Like my little half-Jewish pupil he seemed ideally nordic. When I knew many years later of the stand he had made against the domination of the Nazis, my sadness at his death was partially eased by gladness that he had not deceived me; that he was the man I thought he was. Some people have said that Karl Haushofer, his father, wrote *Mein Kampf*.

Hitler was in prison and Hess had taken refuge with the Haushofers. I wonder if I ever met him. I knew nothing of the German politics of the day and if I had encountered him in that hospitable house I would not have been impressed. With Hitler temporarily out of the way, visited daily, as I learned later, by Karl Haushofer, Munich was quiet. Only once was my own peace disturbed.

Years after it happened I went back to Munich and tried to find the street, but I couldn't. I couldn't find one anything like it. Perhaps it had got mixed in my mind with others I knew then, for it seems to me that it was like a Pimlico street, long and straight and porticoed, with a splash of green in the distance where it ended in St George's Square cr Grosvenor Road.

The street was full of sunshine. The sun shone on the yellow houses and cast black shadows in the porticos and glinted in the leaves of the distant trees. It was an evening for a stroll or for lounging and talking to the neighbours. I knew at once that there was something strange about it, but I had walked twenty yards down it, thinking about something else, before I realized what it was. There was no one in it, except for me on the pavement and a big fair young man who walked in the middle of the road ahead of me.

I didn't like it, but there was no reason for turning back. The other man didn't like it either. His legs wanted to run but he wouldn't let them. I could see his neck muscles taut with the effort not to look round. So we went on along the street towards the trees at the end which reminded me of the three silver birches which were always 'home' when we played hide-and-seek in my uncle's garden at Harston. To get to them you had to cross a great open stretch of lawn without cover, so you sprinted the last fifty yards. A grown-up man can't suddenly start sprinting in broad daylight in a respectable residential street in a great city.

The other man wasn't worrying about me. Once he relaxed and looked round and caught my eye. He was frightened but not of me. He thought we were in the same boat, but what boat I didn't know. He almost signalled 'Shall we run?' but thought better of it, resumed his dignity, and went on walking very fast towards the green trees.

Then a rifle cracked and he was lying in the road. Almost before his face crashed into the hot asphalt I was in the nearest portico. He lay there in the sun with a red puddle forming slowly round his head, while nothing happened. There was no man with a rifle, no policeman, no staring crowd. No window opened. In the silence which came when our footsteps and the echoes of the shot had ceased, you could hear the murmur of traffic and the hooting of taxi horns in nearby streets. In our street there was nothing, except the sunshine and myself crouching in a doorway and a dead man in the road.

Nothing went on happening and became tedious. So I went away. Keeping very close to the houses, I gained the trees.

They weren't birch trees at all. I was excited now and a little pleased with myself, but at the general's house the story didn't go down at all well. You never knew what would happen in a decent city when damned Austrian house painters were allowed to play old Harry with the place. It was a bad thing for foreigners to get mixed up in these things. No it would not be wise to go to the police. Forget all about it. Don't tell anyone. People who know too much. . . . That made me laugh. I wanted to know a lot more, but he wouldn't go on talking about it.

In the circumstances of 1923, with the mark sliding rapidly into the abyss, I was pleasantly rich. I still have the excellent Goertz camera that I bought for sixpence. I could afford on my days off to climb with guides, a thing impossible for me in Switzerland, and the valley of Garmisch lay at the very foot of the Wettersteingebirge.

The valley was wide and very fertile, at one end opening out into the flat Bavarian plain, at the other narrowing to a deep defile, the Höllenthal, which led tortuously, lit by sunshine at noonday only, deep into the little range of the Wetterstein, a crescent of sharp peaks on the Austrian frontier. It had not then become a fashionable resort and the village at the valley's head was still small, a cluster of brightly coloured ancient houses and a single white hotel. Outside the Post Hotel the local guides whiled away the halcyon summer of 1923 in a philosophical haze of smoke, earning occasionally a very small fee for escorting a middle-aged couple along the path through the Höllenthal, the Devil's Valley. Amongst them even the strangers from Munich could recognize Georg Scheurrer, whose handsome bearded face decorated the windows of picture-postcard shops even in the distant capital.

Scheurrer was unknown outside southern Germany but there he was supreme amongst the guides. A sure, steady, rhythmical climber on the steepest rock faces, a tireless leader on ice and snow whose strength seemed infinite and whose judgement never failed, he emanated an aura of kindliness, trust and quiet humour which seemed a distillation of the mountain peace of his upland valley. In the years to come when I was sometimes tempted to believe the old soldiers' saying 'The only good Germans are dead Germans', I would remember him.

That summer Scheurrer, pleased to find an experienced companion, climbed with me; or, temporarily an amateur, with his friend Simon Maurer, a fine climber too but mentally a peasant like the rest, kindly but insensitive, religious but superstitious. In winter Scheurrer taught me to ski. As a performer he was superb, delighting in tricks which in that valley only he could play.

In the autumn of 1923, my hostess, Scheurrer, Maurer and I celebrated the end of a perfect summer with a three-day expedition farther afield than the little peaks of the Wetterstein. On the second day we climbed the Südwand of the Musterstein and on the third Maurer and I left the other two to less ambitious schemes and made for the Dreitorspitze. The steep eastern side of the mountain, the Ostkante, had only once been ascended and on that occasion the leader, Dr Donnermann, had assisted his ascent by the use of pitons hammered into the rock. It was rumoured in the valley that means even more unsporting had been used, but a curious silence fell upon the company whenever I tried to learn the details of the story. Even Maurer, Donnermann's companion on the first ascent, refused to talk. Only one thing emerged, that he didn't 'count' the first ascent because of the pitons and that he had been waiting impatiently for a suitable companion to climb the huge face of rock a second time and without artificial aids.

For three hours Maurer led quietly and steadily. Run-outs of a hundred feet of rope were sometimes necessary before he could reach a point of comparative safety to which I too could climb. The whole face was continuously steep and difficult, and in places awe-inspiring, but Maurer never paused for longer than was necessary to shepherd me to each insufficient stance. As time passed I began to long for just one pause between stepping gingerly from hold to tiny hold and between the anxious minutes in which I paid out the rope to a steadily climbing leader whose life at any moment might depend upon my watchfulness. I longed for two minutes to eat a stick of chocolate or take a pull at my water-bottle or relight my pipe. But even on the stances

on which Simon and I momentarily stood together one had to
hang on with at least one hand and the space was so cramped
that I had no sooner secured my rope that he would be moving on
again. But the sky remained, as it had been for months, an uninterrupted blue and the autumn sun shone steadily warming
the rocks and our hearts, and even the longing for a pause was
stilled by the exaltation of that glorious climb.

Then suddenly we were there, lying on the close-cropped turf
of the summit and before us a delightful run, unroped, down
easy rock to lunch at the hut. But before we left the summit,
lying there sucking at our pipes, relaxed and happy in our achieve-
ment, I heard another bit of the Donnermann story.

'Today' said Maurer, 'we have really climbed the Ostkante.'

'The second time for you,' I said.

'But this time, I led.'

'And beautifully. I am sure Donnermann didn't lead like that.
Anyway, he used pitons.'

'Donnermann' said Maurer, 'did not always lead. I never saw
who did. You remember that corner we went round on our
bellies? When you could not see me for a hundred feet? I heard
Donnermann talking there as though to a friend and I heard
someone answer, but I couldn't hear what was said. But he
climbed that difficult hundred feet in a matter of seconds and
from that time he climbed as though he were second on the
rope, paying out a rope I could not see to someone he was
watching ahead of him, before taking in my rope and bringing
me up to his stance. And when I asked him about it he laughed at
me and called me an ignorant peasant.'

At the hut, Scheurrer was still 'cagey'. You could rarely make
him suggest anything unkind about anybody. But he reminded
me of the time when he had led a girl and myself up the Sonnenspitzl, and she, unable to reach a hand-hold, had stood on my
head and had there become hysterical, stamping her nailed boots
on my scalp and crying that she could go no farther. He had
seen the same thing happen with Donnermann, and he had
said something quietly in a language Scheurrer could not understand and for the rest of that day the girl had climbed beautifully

and confidently, and afterwards had remembered nothing of it.

It was months later, on the long cliff above the Sonnenspitzl that Scheurrer talked again. We had come on skis up the long slopes from the Rainthal and were resting in the snow before crashing down again. And this was the story he told me.

Donnermann was (is, for all I know) a psychiatrist in a city not far from the Wetterstein. He used hypnotism and in consequence gained a somewhat sinister reputation which was only partially off-set by his extraordinary skill as a climber and skier. Indeed there were those who said that his prowess was not altogether of this world. He seems to have had a remarkable personality and a special power of influencing women. His nurse-receptionist adored him and he rewarded her devotion to an extent which annoyed his wife into a threat of divorce proceedings. In a largely Catholic community, such a threat was a serious one to a professional man. He dismissed his nurse but continued to meet her in the mountains. His wife discovered this and consulted her lawyer. Donnermann promised to break finally with his mistress, but this was not easy. She was a strong-minded girl and very much in love. Donnermann saw his lucrative practice in imminent danger.

It was at this point in the story that the girl died, and we have no information except what Donnermann gave to the police. He said that late one evening he had a telephone call from her. She said she was in the Wetterstein mountains and that she had decided to have a fatal accident unless he promised, there and then, that he would leave his wife and come to her. He was a psychiatrist, and he knew that she meant what she said. He did the only possible thing in the circumstances, gave the promise (which, he said later, he did not intend to keep) and set off in pursuit, with the object of talking to her and inducing her to be reasonable.

He knew the country perfectly and there was a full moon. In the morning he arrived at the hut, to find that she had left. He followed her tracks upwards, by now in fear that she had seen through his deception and had decided to carry out her original plan. After a long trudge he saw her ahead of him, increased his

pace and caught up with her a few hundred feet below the top
of the long line of cliffs which look down upon the valley of the
Loisach. Here they talked, at first quietly, but as time passed
more and more emotionally, until finally she broke away from
him. There was a struggle in the snow. She was fit, and fresh
from a night's rest in the hut. He was unfit from too little exercise of late and had skied all night to reach her. In the struggle he
slipped, and as he fell his head crashed against a rock and he lost
consciousness. When he recovered, one set of tracks led from
where he lay to the cliff edge, and the girl had gone. That was
his story.

The police, of course, came at once and examined the snow
before another fall could obscure the evidence. Suicide was the
obvious conclusion and Donnermann, whose earlier peccadilloes
were conveniently whitewashed, came rather well out of the adventure.

'Well,' I said, 'I think he did. He seems to have done his best,
at any rate at the end of the story.'

'It looks like it,' said Scheurrer. 'There was only one set of
tracks from the spot where we are sitting now, the place where
the struggle happened, and Donnermann hit his head and was
stunned – one set to the edge of the cliff and no returning tracks.
Only one person could have gone up to the edge and that one did
not return. They were the deep tracks of a skier with a heavy
load, but what of that? She had gone out equipped for a three-
day skilauf. Curious that she didn't leave her rucksack at the
hut, but anyway she didn't; Donnermann said so.'

'I will show you,' said Scheurrer, 'just where she must have
gone over.'

He started towards the cliff, up the gentle slope towards the
edge. I noticed that he wasn't herring-boning as was his habit.
Gradually slowly and carefully he neared the edge, reached it,
hesitated for a moment. Suddenly he turned and shot down
towards me. From where I stood one set of tracks ascended to
the skyline.

In 1924 the meteorologist who lived in a hut on the top of the

Zugspitze at about 3,000 metres was alone from the autumn, when the last climbers went, until the spring when the first skiers came. He seemed happy with the Bible and the transactions of the various scientific societies to which he belonged, but his friend Kiliani, an electrical engineer, thought that he should move with the times and have a radio, and I was enlisted to help. All would probably have been well if Kiliani had had any aesthetic sense. On September 23rd he unfortunately fell in with a girl whom he described in rapturous terms and invited to join us. She was fat and pale and reminded me of nothing more endearing than a young pig.

So at seven in the morning we set out, heavily burdened, for in those days receiving sets were very large and heavy, to climb the Zugspitze by the long walk up the Rainthal and the Partnachklam. Up the easy valley slopes we made good progress and, despite our loads, we reached the Angerhütte at midday and rested there for an hour.

It was then that things began to go wrong. The faultless sky became cloudy and the steps of the piglet slower and more uncertain. The path became steeper and rougher, and our progress up the 700 feet to the Knorrhütte woefully slow; it took two hours. By that time, massive clouds were building up over the Austrian frontier and the piglet decided to demonstrate British courage. 'We must go on,' she said. We relieved her of her small load and raced the clouds, which won easily. It is only 900 feet from the Knorrhütte to the summit and in daylight an easy climb, every slightly difficult pitch thoughtfully draped with ladders and steel ropes. The piglet again decided to demonstrate British courage. At intervals she stopped and sat down upon the soft thick cushion with which Nature had liberally endowed her. 'Go on,' she said, 'and leave me here. I will not be responsible for your deaths.' By that time it was very dark and we had no light, for we had expected to reach the top by six o'clock. Kiliani and I took it in turns to go ahead and reconnoitre the route, and then return to guide the other who carried on his shoulders not only his share of the receiving set but also the unlovely burden of the piglet.

At last we saw a lighted window above us, and the meteorologist with a torch came to our call. It was about ten o'clock, and we spent a pleasant evening drinking the local liqueur, *Enzian*, and listening to a broadcast from the Savoy Orpheans in London, the first time the lovely silence of the Wettersteingebirge had been so polluted.

The next day the piglet was heard to remark that she had enjoyed herself so much that she thought she would like to take up climbing. Kiliani, still apparently entranced, agreed to take her home over the Waxensteins. I bid them a hurried farewell, and dropped alone down the northern side of the Zugspitze to a rapturous bathe in the Eibsee and a bus to Garmisch. I never saw either of my companions again.

Frau Mayer and Hanno had invited me to go back to Garmisch in January 1924, not this time as tutor but as friend. A perfect winter followed a perfect summer. The snow was so thick that we put on our skis in the front hall, and slid down the invisible steps into the garden and away between the high banks of snow to the practice slopes. We had Scheurrer's undivided attention from breakfast-time till the light failed and in the evenings danced at the Post Hotel to the local band, for she had abandoned her widow's weeds.

But term-time was approaching. Scheurrer was pleased enough with our progress to suggest a mountain trip, a skilauf, but there was no time and I had to refuse. Frau Mayer came to the rescue. If I would stay she would pay for me to fly from Cologne to London. We had our mountain trip.

It was a curious time in Germany. In Bavaria, where the Prussians were not liked, there was a powerful faction in favour of separation and a renewal of the old kingdom under the able charming (but happily unambitious) Prince Ruprecht, the heir to the old monarchy. I first realized this when I stood in an egg queue behind an obvious Prussian. The egg woman would have none of him. 'I will not sell eggs to a foreigner!' My turn was next and I approached with diffidence. '*Ach, ein Englander.* Welcome! How many eggs?'

Meanwhile an official boundary had been created between Bavaria and the rest of Germany.

My passport was, I thought, in order and I had a German visa. At Aschaffenburg, however, trouble arose. This was the border between Bavaria and the rest of the Reich, and I had no entry permit into Bavaria. It therefore followed that I couldn't leave for I had not officially entered. After much argument I was taken off the train, which continued, with my luggage, to Cologne, and was conducted by two policemen, heavily armed, through the snowy streets to a huge red stone castle and a mediaeval dungeon. The only furniture was a wooden bench and I spent the night on the stone floor, reading Dakin's *Oxidations and Reductions in the Animal Body*. I was given no food and felt reduction was the more appropriate word of the two. Next morning I appeared before a magistrate. Somebody had arranged for me to be represented by counsel. I understood almost nothing of what went on. Everybody got very angry and the two counsel shouted at each other over my uncomprehending head, till suddenly quiet came. The magistrate rose, descended, walked to the dock, shook me by the hand and I was free.

I was, of course, a day late. At Cologne I stayed the night at the Dom Hotel, found my luggage, and asked about my route. The aeroplane had gone the day before and there would not be another for several more days. Trains to Ostend for civilians were few and slow, but there would be a fast military train that afternoon. A special pass was needed, to be obtained only from the transport officer of the British army of occupation. Ex-Lance-Corporal Greene, temporarily self-promoted to the rank of Second Lieutenant in the Hertfordshire Regiment, got his pass, but it was an embarrassing journey.

It was only twelve years before I saw Garmisch again, but the alpine village had become a tourist centre. It had grown so much that I couldn't find the Villa Lützenkirchen. Nobody had heard of the Mayers or of Scheurrer or of Maurer. Rumours had reached me and I did not try to find the Haushofers. Only the Wettersteingebirge were unchanged.

3 The Beast 666

In 1922 I had never heard of Aleister Crowley. In November of that year *John Bull*, a much-read weekly edited by the infamous Horatio Bottomley, began a highly coloured 'exposure' of this 'foul and blasphemous propagandist'. Reading it again I can re-experience the laughter and excitement the articles aroused in me. I had already begun to look on Black Magic as a subject of hilarious psychological interest.

Crowley had, said *John Bull*, published many books 'distinguished for their wild, erotic, blasphemous and disgusting imagery'. Some of them I read; they would seem to the modern reader very tame and unintentionally funny, the product of a mind deranged and immature. He was said, with some justice, to be the promoter of a mission to attract weak-minded people of both sexes to the teaching of mediaeval alchemists and magicians, with the additional attractions of barbaric and licentious orgies conducted amidst clouds of incense in a darkened room. I was a little stopped in my laughter by the discovery that General J. F. C. Fuller, the greatest military strategist of his day, was not only an admirer of Crowley but had also written a book about him called *The Star in the West*. But my sense of the ridiculous overcame even this discovery. According to *John Bull*, Crowley had spent the first Great War conducting violent pro-German propaganda in the U.S.A. Later, in my delighted tongue-in-cheek investigations, I found evidence that he had been throughout a very successful *agent provocateur* whose communications to the British secret service had been of some value in disclosing many anti-British 'cells' that were promptly destroyed when America entered the war.

Another discovery worried me as a keen young climber. Crowley had been a very expert mountaineer who had climbed with some of the most distinguished alpinists of that time and had organized a Himalayan expedition, from which, it must be admitted, he had emerged with little credit.

The *Sunday Express* took up the hue and cry. Its investigations showed, to its own satisfaction, that he had organized societies for pagan orgies; had engaged in pro-German propaganda during the war; had published obscene attacks on the King; had renounced his British nationality; had supported the Irish rebels and had proclaimed himself 'King of Ireland' (an accusation that didn't make the *Sunday Express* laugh!); had stolen money from a woman (a woman!); and was now the head of an 'abbey in Sicily' where obscene magical and sexual rites were the order of the day.

Up to this time I regarded Crowley as a psychologically interesting and altogether laughable 'case'. But in February 1923 I was suddenly forced to straighten my face. Walking into the lodge of Pembroke College, I was faced by a copy of the *Sunday Express* that announced 'More Sinister Revelations of Aleister Crowley. Varsity Lad's Death. Dreadful Ordeal of a Young Wife.' My friend, Raoul Loveday, had died mysteriously at the Collegium ad Spiritum Sanctum at Cefalu in Sicily. Raoul, according to the *Sunday Express*, had married 'a beautiful girl prominent in London artistic circles' who had arrived home in a state of collapse, 'unable to give more than a hint of the horrors from which she has escaped'. The *Sunday Express* had no difficulty in expanding this 'hint' into many columns in this and future issues. Although 'the facts are too unutterably filthy to be detailed in a newspaper, for they have to do with sexual orgies that touch the lowest depths of depravity', and although 'the beautiful young wife' had been unable to give more than a hint of what went on, the paper did indeed give enough detail to raise its sales in Oxford to considerable levels.

Raoul Loveday had been a small, fair man whose interests were divided between football, at which he was very good, and the construction of remarkably bad poetry. In his later Oxford days he had suddenly developed a passionate interest in black magic. He was suspected of taking drugs but I think he fostered the rumour. If he used them it was probably only occasionally and out of curiosity; certainly I never saw him in a drugged state. His extra curricular activities made serious work impossible, and he narrowly escaped being sent down from St John's. Shortly afterwards he electrified and infuriated the Senior Common Room by getting a first class in history. I was not one of his most intimate friends, but not even these knew anything of his origins. He was vaguely supposed to be the son of a retired naval officer who had become a King's Messenger. It was not till he was dead that I found that his father was in fact a retired naval officer, but a petty officer, and that the 'King' for whom he ran messages was my uncle, Sir Graham Greene, who had been Secretary of the Admiralty. My uncle described him as a 'very decent dependable fellow'. It was only after Raoul's death that I learned that he had gone to Sicily to be 'secretary' to Crowley, having in the meantime married Betty May, an artists' model, known in two artistic circles anyway, the Fitzroy Tavern in Windmill Street and the Harlequin Club in Soho, neither then very salubrious haunts.

Afterwards I met her. She was in bed at the Golden Cross Hotel in Oxford, holding court to Raoul's friends, and to any others who might be useful in her journalistic campaign. She was, I guessed, in the early thirties and very attractive in a rare Mongolian way. One could understand why Jacob Epstein had used her as a model. She showed no signs of shock and her description of the Abbey at Cefalu was singularly detailed and devoid of hints. On arrival they had had a long dreary climb up a muddy mountainous path until the Abbey loomed up suddenly before them, the white walls gleaming eerily in the faint moon-light, one mysterious flickering light shining from a small window. There they were forced to take part in terrible rites and orgies until Raoul became mysteriously ill, according to her because of drugs administered against his will. When he died she wandered all night in the lonely hills (a rather unnecessary activity, five minutes' walk from a reasonably good hotel) and finally escaped by the skin of her teeth and the intervention of the British Consul.

Throughout 1923 the *Sunday Express* and *John Bull* continued their violent and certainly libellous attacks. The undergraduate world of Oxford was thrilled to the marrow. Peter Rodd, son of the British Ambassador in Rome, came with a friend, now a member of the House of Lords, to my rooms with the proposal that I should go to Cefalu, shoot Crowley and make my way across the mountains to the south coast of Sicily. Here he and his friend would meet me in a sailing boat and take me across the Mediterranean to the north coast of Africa, whence I could make my escape by way of Morocco, Gibraltar and Spain. Peter's friend would pay all expenses. My reply was disappointing; I had no proof that Crowley deserved death and felt that the evidence of Betty May was of doubtful validity; I had no wish to spend an indefinite time in an Italian gaol, or even die there; and my only reason for believing that Peter was a competent navigator was that he had coxed the Balliol second 'togger'. He never really believed that I had turned down his scheme, and told several people that I was bent on following it. I have still a very pompous letter from Richard Hughes, another friend of Raoul's, who has become a famous writer, strongly advising me against pushing my nose into what did not concern me, a letter that I remembered with a chuckle when I later met 'Dickon' in Sicily, also on the hunt for Crowley.

Though I was not willing to join any hare-brained scheme, I was full of curiosity, and when the Easter vacation of 1923 arrived I decided to go to Sicily.

The final decision was forced upon me by Crowley who, at this time, I had never met.

'Dear Sir,' he wrote. 'Do what thou wilt shall be the Whole of the Law. Forgive me if I suggest, from the little experience that I have in such matters, that when one is establishing a spy system it is rather important to prevent one's principal plan coming directly into the hands of the person whom you want watched . . . Love is the law, love under will. Yours truly, Aleister Crowley, Knight Guardian of the Sangraal.'

Claud Bosanquet, a young don of Christ Church and a climbing friend, decided to come with me to have a look at the mountains there. The loose tongue of Peter Rodd had not gone unheard. A friend who stayed on at the Park Hotel in Rome after our departure later told us that the police had made inquiries for us there. They were told that we had gone to the Hotel de France at Palermo, and we later learned that inquiries were indeed made by the police there, again too late. They then lost the trail.

At Palermo an incident occurred that was later exaggerated by Louis Golding in his novel *The Camberwell Beauty*, in which young Webster, whom I can hardly recognize as myself, was kidnapped by the Mafia. In fact I was alone at a puppet show, and in the dark I began to realize that a group of rather sinister men was beginning gradually, as the earlier occupants left, to occupy the seats around me. I was beginning to feel a little nervous and to tell myself not to be so foolish, when a man behind me leant forward till his mouth was near my ear and whispered, in unaccented English, 'Get out quick!' . . . I did. Using the techniques of a rugger player, I reached the door. In the sunshine outside a group of policemen lazed and chatted. The pursuit ended and I strolled away. My further adventures in *The Camberwell Beauty* are wholly fictitious.

Nevertheless Bosanquet and I thought that it would be injudicious to wander through Sicily with more than a minimum of money. I handed him my spare cash and he deposited it with his own at the reception desk. Then we left for Cefalu.

Cefalu is forty miles from Palermo, a large village with a railway station, a hotel and a force of carabinieri. Our inquiries suggested that Crowley was quite well-liked and certainly not feared. The sinister 'abbey' of Betty May and the journalists was a small white bungalow, surrounded by olive trees about five minutes' walk above the village. As we approached we could hear the laughter of children. They were clean and healthy and did not seem to have been upset by having been, as *John Bull* had said, 'forced to witness nameless horrors'. They were called Hermes, Dionysus and Astarte Lulu Panthea. They were undoubtedly Crowley's children, but I was never sure which of his female disciples had mothered them. Crowley was absent. Knowing by his 'magical intuition' (supported as I found later by a sight of letters addressed to me at the poste restante) that I was on my way, he had delayed his necessary departure to Naples, but had finally been forced to go, accompanied by his 'secretary' Miss Helsig, alias Countess Harcourt, alias Lea, alias the Scarlet Woman, alias the Virgin (*sic*) Guardian of the Sangraal, alias Alostrael, hereafter known as Alostrael. Alostrael, we were told, was not to go all the way to Naples, but would await his return at the Savoy Hotel in Palermo.

The living-room was large and untidy but full of sunshine and smelling slightly of incense. On the stone floor were painted triangles and pentacles and interlacing circles, and on the walls were many very crude paintings by The Beast. In the bookshelf were books on magic, many by Crowley himself. On that occasion we were shown no more, but returned to Palermo.

We took rooms at the Savoy Hotel, where I had no difficulty in being introduced to Alostrael, a pretty, thin woman in the middle thirties, with a very excitable manner. Seeing her now, I would have guessed her to be under the influence of amphetamine, but this drug had not then been invented. Till a late hour she expounded with great enthusiasm the doctrines of The Beast.

Next day, John Pilley, 'Dickon' Hughes and Peter Quennell arrived on the scene. I left Bosanquet with them and returned with Alostrael to Cefalu. This time I was allowed to see 'la chambre des cauchemars', a small room whose walls were covered with crude paintings of such obscenity that I had difficulty in preserving the gravity to be expected of one being initiated into a new religion.

I left convinced that Raoul had died a natural death, and Dr Maggio, an obviously reliable man who had attended him, confirmed this. I returned relieved to Palermo, rejoined my friends, and spent a day climbing with them on the Pizzo del Carne above Altavilla. That evening Hughes, Quennell and Pilley decided to spend the night on the mountain, and Bosanquet, who mistrusted their capacity to look after themselves, stayed with them. I, less conscientious than Bosanquet and aware to what depths the temperature in April may drop at night, even in the far south of Europe, descended the mountainside to the railway and returned to Palermo and the Hotel de France.

The next morning I was due to begin my return journey, intending to break it at Naples where I had been told to look for Crowley at Michaelson's bookshop. I therefore asked the manager for my money. He looked at me suspiciously.

'What money?'

'The money Mr Bosanquet and I left with you.'

'Certainly Mr Bosanquet left money with me and I gave him a receipt.'

'Half of that was mine.'

'How do I know that? Where is your receipt? Believe me, sir, I do not really disbelieve you, but you must see that without Mr Bosanquet's permission I cannot give you any of the money he left in my charge. And where is Mr Bosanquet?'

'For all I know he is frozen stiff on the summit of the Pizzo del Carne. I have only three *lire*. How on earth can I settle your bill and get home to England?'

'As to my bill, leave with me a note to Mr Bosanquet asking him to pay me. As to your return, I would advise you to consult the British Consul.'

Frederick Gambier MacBean, his Britannic Majesty's Consul in Palermo, was a small, unsmiling Scot who listened to my story and then expressed at great length his detestation of irresponsible undergraduates. He refused to lend me any money. I suggested that he might send a telegram to my father, but he had no funds earmarked for such a purpose. I threatened to throw myself on the mercy of the police as a vagrant without visible means of support. This shook him a little and after another diatribe he sent a clerk with me to the station with instructions to buy me a third class ticket to London, but to give me no cash. I started the long journey with my three *lire* still intact.

At Michaelson's bookshop they told me that Crowley was in Taormina, which I did not believe. I crossed the road to Thomas Cook, and was inquiring if they knew the whereabouts of Mr Aleister Crowley, when a voice behind me chanted, 'Do what thou wilt shall be the Whole of the Law,' and I turned and introduced myself. He was a big man of forty-seven, inclined to be corpulent, with a bald head, grey hair and a sallow complexion. His figure drooped and he had a dragging gait. His manner was peevish and he had a slight cockney accent. He was not my idea of a magician and seemed disappointingly unsinister.

I spent the morning with him and had a good lunch which, thanks to Frederick Gambier MacBean, I greatly enjoyed. I was far from impressed by the great magician's mental powers. For a long time he would not leave the subject of rock-climbing. When finally I got him to talk about drugs and sex, he seemed rather bored. Drugs, he believed, are only dangerous to those who fear them; the wise man uses heroin or opium or cocaine as he uses alcohol or nicotine. Ether perhaps pleased him most; it was possible to get drunk and sober again several times a day. As to sex, copulate freely by all means, but don't get too emotional about it; the emotion of love destroys the intellect.

He was immensely conceited. I asked him why he didn't sue the papers which so vilely maligned him. 'I am', he said, 'great enough to ignore public opinion. Did Shelley bring libel actions? No, he came to Italy. Did Byron bring libel actions? No, he came to Italy. Did I bring libel actions? No, I have come to Italy.' But years later he went back on these words.

I saw Crowley again occasionally over the next twenty years. He never again achieved the notoriety of 1923. He continued to write poems and occult books that nobody read but that now are valuable collectors' pieces. I don't think he was 'The Wickedest Man in the World' as the journalist 'Cassandra' called him. He was a very silly man and I doubt whether he did anybody any real harm.

I was, at twenty-two, far too shy to borrow money from him and so, still with three *lire* in my pocket, I boarded the train to Rome. The third-class carriage was almost filled with peculiarly odorous and apparently villainous men, the exception being a very young and pretty fair-haired girl, who was obviously in great distress. Noticing that she was reading an English novel,

I asked her whether I could help her. She told me that she was Swiss and had been with her husband in Naples. She wanted to go to Capri, but her husband, who knew the island well, preferred to explore Naples, so she went alone, arranging to meet him on her return. He was not at the station and she panicked. She succeeded in getting herself and her luggage aboard, thinking only of rejoining her family in Rome, but there her courage failed. The thought of removing her luggage and herself from the train and reaching the hotel was more than she could face. At Rome I took her under my wing, refused the services of a porter, found a cab and drove her to her hotel, wondering how I could pay the driver. At the hotel a porter opened the door of the cab and took charge of her luggage. I told him in a lordly way to pay the driver, and was about to escape when she seized me by the arm crying, 'No, you cannot leave me yet. They may not be here.' They were, a large and friendly Swiss family who, after a moment of justifiable suspicion, decided that I was Sir Galahad. I ate well, knowing that it might be my last meal for many hours. After dinner her father took me to the station, settled me in my compartment and disappeared. He returned a few minutes later with a vast basket of food and a bottle of wine. I ate well all the way to England, and arrived at Victoria with my three *lire* intact.

Crowley died in obscurity in 1947, and the journalist 'Cassandra' went to his funeral in the crematorium at Hastings. 'Crowley, this strange old man, this dubious artist in necromantic mumbo-jumbo, who had founded an iniquitous abbey in Sicily, had been expelled from France, banned in England, and entangled in a series of ferocious and disreputable lawsuits, had come to the end of the road. An elderly man stepped up to what passes for a pulpit in a crematorium. . . . In a deep loud voice of considerable eloquence he began to read A Hymn to Pan:

"Oh Pan! Pan! Pan! Satan has come on a Milk White Ass. . . . The Great Beast has come. . . . I am in the grip of the snake. . . . O Pan! O Pan! O Pan! I am borne to Death on the

26

Horns of the unicorn. O Pan! Pan! Pan! Do what thou wilt shall be the Whole of the Law. Love is the Law, love under will." '

The Knight Guardian of the Sangraal was silly, even in death.

The story has another sequel. During the war I was attached to the Emergency Hospital at Aylesbury. Someone asked me to tell the Crowley Saga, which I did, including the incident of Frederick Gambier MacBean.

'Why,' asked the very attractive anaesthetist, 'didn't you put a curse on him? You must have learnt a few good curses at the Abbey.'

'It never occurred to me,' I replied, 'but I will do it now.'

I made up a long and resounding curse, partly out of the nonsensical rituals of the Crowley sect and partly from my own imagination. Two days later I found the anaesthetist staring with troubled eyes at the front page of *The Times* spread out on the table. Frederick Gambier MacBean was dead.

4 Morocco Then and Now

I first went to Morocco in 1928. The Riff War was hardly over, but in Tangier everything seemed peaceful. I wanted to go farther afield. Walter Harris, the witty and learned correspondent of *The Times*, sent me to Fez. 'I have', he said, 'been to every oriental city you can name, but for me Fez is still the epitome of the East.'

On the platform of a railway station where I had to change my train, I saw a familiar figure, that of Jim Wyllie, an artist who ran a restaurant, the Moorish Café, in Oxford. We had never been introduced and so, of course, were hesitant about committing the impertinence of addressing each other. We had a long time to wait and suddenly our British reticence collapsed and simultaneously we greeted each other. He has been one of my closest friends ever since and is the godfather of my son.

Jim had originally gone to Morocco with a view to learning Arabic and joining the Foreign Office. He did the first but not the second. He nearly led me into buying with him a little house in the Kasbah of Tangier that was going for a song. Hugh Gurney, the Consul-General, aided and abetted him, promising me that every foreigner in Morocco would seek my advice. I resisted with difficulty. Jim bought the house, added the adjoining houses and has lived there ever since except for short terms in the summer at the Portmeirion Hotel in North Wales, of which he was manager for a time and remains a director.

With him I explored Fez, which was everything Walter Harris had said, a jewel of an ancient eastern city, unspoiled by modernity. I was told that Lyautey, the French Governor of Morocco, had found his French subjects beginning to demolish

28

the old city and replacing it by modern French architecture, always (till Corbusier) the worst in the world. He took an immediate decision to pull down all new work and to found a new Fez, far enough away to leave the old city unspoiled.

In Tangier, Jim knew a rich and entertaining Moor named Monty Corcos, who had served in the Royal Flying Corps in the Kaiser's war and had become very anglophil. We were having a drink with him one evening when he asked how we were travelling, and was stunned to hear that we used trains and buses. 'You *must*,' he said, 'have one of my cars.' Out of five or six we chose a dependable-looking Buick, and the next day set out to cover the few miles along what was then hardly better than a track between Tangier and Tetuan. Monty impressed upon us that we must not linger near the side-road that led to Xauen. Though peace had officially been declared, the Riffs in this their sacred city had a regrettable tendency to descend from their fastness in the mountains and kidnap any hapless Europeans whose cars had broken down on the main 'road', thereafter sending their fingers, one by one, to their appropriate consuls in Tangier with demands for ransom.

Needless to say, we broke down at the crucial point. We knew nothing about the insides of motor cars and were helpless. We had not seen a car since leaving Tangier, but within an hour the road, which was only wide enough for one, was blocked fore and aft by many motors, the owners of which, more I think from terror than from kindness, were trying unsuccessfully to help us.

Suddenly there arrived the *deus ex machina*. The *deus* was a cockney chauffeur and the *machina* a Rolls-Royce. He looked at us suspiciously and asked what we were doing with Mr Corcos's car. Accepting our explanation, he said, 'I used to be Mr Corcos's chauffeur. This always 'appened to this bloody Buick. I know what's wrong.' He unscrewed the petrol lead, sucked out about half a pint of petrol, spat it in the face of a neighouring 'wog', started the car again, refused a tip and, with the expertise of a London policeman, sorted out the traffic. We drove without further incident to Tetuan.

This was in 1928. Seven years later my bride and I travelled
by that road, now smooth and much more straight, and took the
road to Xauen itself, where we stayed in a somewhat inferior
hotel. There was deep snow on the ground, enhancing the beauty
of an already lovely little town. There was no central or indeed
any other heating, the architect being firmly of the belief that
any part of the world south of Spain was permanently tropical.
There was running water in our bedroom, but both H. and C.
taps ran icy cold. However, the sherry was good.

Another twenty years passed and we returned. Now there is a
luxurious hotel and excellent food. But I think Xauen was more
fun in 1928.

From Tangier, Jim and I went to Casablanca, an unlovely
town, on our way to Marrakech. In those days an ancient Ford,
with a body like the covered wagon of a wild western film, took
the best part of a day to vibrate and boil its uneasy way over the
stony downland which lies between Casablanca and the ancient
capital. Just as all hope of arrival began to evaporate in the
clouds of steam from the rusty radiator, the 'bus' topped the
rise and, surrounded by green fields, the low red city of Marrakech el Hamah lay lovely at one's feet, the tall green finger of the
Kutubiah outlined against the white snows of Atlas.

It was early summer but the heat in the south had already
dried the red dust in which the beggars sat and demonstrated,
to the few who stopped to look, their sores and mutilations. The
tables set, also in the dust, outside the little café were filled. I
had just, after prolonged and lazy contemplation of a nearby
beggar, arrived by a process of elimination at the conclusion that
his disease was certainly self-inflicted, when I became aware of
a strange figure at the next table. Clad in that stuffy heat in the
seedy but conventional dress of a London businessman, varied
by the strange addition of a straw boater at one end and a pair
of brown buttoned boots at the other, sat a thin, grey-haired
man, accompanied only by a live white rabbit in a brown paper
bag. A row of empty beer bottles grew steadily longer on the
little table before him. Now and again the rabbit wriggled and a
bottle fell with a dull thud into the dust. The man in the

boater picked it up and replaced it meticulously in line. Then he cuffed the rabbit.

My own collection of bottles, less tidily arranged, grew as fast, and with it grew my curiosity until at last it overcame the inhibitions of the Englishman abroad. I took my glass in my hand and sitting firmly opposite him demanded enlightenment.

'Why' I said, 'do you carry about with you a white rabbit in a brown paper bag?' For a full half minute he regarded me solemnly and then, neglecting my question, spoke.

'Good morning, doctor,' he said, 'we have met before.' I confessed apologetically that I had no memory of a previous meeting. 'In Malaya,' he said.

'I have never been to Malaya.'

'But you are a doctor?'

'Yes.'

'A pathologist?'

'No.'

'A most curious resemblance.' He went on. 'I remember your double so very clearly. I am most unlikely, really, ever to forget him, not because he was in any way remarkable in appearance' (I bowed politely), 'but because of the circumstances, which were really so *very* remarkable.'

He was set on telling me his story and I, with a morning to while away, did nothing to discourage him. It appeared that he was the secretary of an important company which owned plantations all over the Far East. One of the Malayan plantations was not doing well. First the output began to fall, then there were discrepancies in the accounts, then letters to the manager were answered belatedly or not at all. Finally, the secretary, whose name, by the way, was Mabbitt ('to rhyme with rabbit', he surprisingly added; and the white rabbit writhed suddenly as though with hidden laughter, and six empty bottles fell off the table), finally, as I say, the secretary was sent out to investigate.

Mabbitt knew all about Malaya. He had gone out there as a small boy with his father who had worked for the same firm, and he had lived there, except for a few years in London, doing his articles till he was forty. He knew everybody there and was already a member of the club in every district. In the club which lay nearest to the unsatisfactory plantation, he settled down to what he thought would be a short and easy job. There was no hurry to begin. He hadn't had leave for a year and he wanted to savour the curiously inverted pleasure of going home to work.

He found that he was not the only recent arrival in the district. There were several doctors living in the club, including the pathologist for whom he had mistaken me. They, too, were investigating a mystery but a rather more difficult one, it appeared. There had been an epidemic of death, a sudden dying for no obvious reason of a large number of apparently healthy natives. The deaths had not been in one district, and there appeared to be nothing to connect them at all. At first nobody took much notice. Registration was not as strict out there as it was in England – it couldn't be with the jungle at your elbow and people appearing and disappearing the whole time, and nobody knowing whether they had died or just skipped over to another valley. Then it became inconvenient and the police got worried. The original sporadic cases became little foci of death. A man would die and then two or three near friends or relations would die too. Then several people near to them would die, and so on. Yet there was no apparent disease. A man would be in the best of health and spirits. Then his father or brother or friend would die. He would look depressed, of course, and maybe weep a little, but he would go on with his work all day, and the next morning he would die. They always died in the morning.

Suddenly everyone began to talk about it. The doctors got busy and did post-mortems on all new cases and even exhumed a few of the old ones, though this wasn't much good, the tropics being what they are. They found nothing to explain the deaths. In the beginning the white settlers, the planters and the official people were worried in case the strange epidemic should attack them, but soon they noticed that the victims were always Malayan – never Indian or European or Chinese. The next thing that was noticed was the singular immunity of children. The youngest patient was eighteen. Men and women suffered about equally. Noticing new facts about the epidemic became a new game in the clubs. On the day Mabbitt arrived, a very pretty girl had just shown that she was intelligent too by pointing out that women with young children were immune. She had been treated by every man in the bar and was still pretty but no longer intelligent.

So my double had been sent for. He was the Professor of Pathology at Singapore and what he didn't know about death in the tropics was nobody's business. He was doing post-mortems at the rate of four a day and he hadn't a clue. The bodies were perfectly healthy and there was no trace of any known poison in them.

They talked of nothing else in the club the night Mabbitt arrived. The argument was chiefly between the people who thought it was a kind of mass hysteria and those who still claimed that it was poison and that the doctors didn't know their job. All the time that he was doing his own investigating, natives went on dying 'like rabbits' (the table heaved suddenly and four more bottles tipped over into the dust). When he had finished his work, he still had several days to spare and he thought he would take a hand in the new game.

Early one morning, when his 'boy' brought him his orange juice and gin, he did something nobody else had thought of doing. He asked his 'boy' what he thought about it. Apparently, to the natives, there was no mystery about it. Life, the 'boy' explained – though naturally he didn't put it quite like that – was a voluntary process. When one no longer wished to live one just died. It was merely necessary to say the right words – tender one's resignation, as one might say – and one just ceased to live. The epidemic? Oh, that too was easily explained. In recent years the natives had become more prosperous and more leisurely. The ties of family affection and of friendship were much stronger. It had happened that several men who were very greatly loved had died and some of their friends had no longer wished to live; and some of their friends too, had found life without them insupportable; and so from those few deaths the ripples had spread throughout the land. Only the grown natives knew the words; the children did not know them; the mothers could not leave their children.

Mabbitt, of course, demanded to know the words. The 'boy' repeated them without hesitation. They were in no language that Mabbitt had ever heard, but he wrote them down phonetically and looked up again, half expecting to see the 'boy' dead on the floor. Instead he was laying out Mabbitt's clothes ready for dressing him. 'I am quite safe,' he explained over his shoulder. 'You see I have just had my breakfast. Food works against the charm. If I had not had breakfast I would have died.'

Mabbitt didn't tell. He couldn't explain why. Several times he started to tell my double but always something stopped him. Perhaps he was afraid of being laughed at, or perhaps he felt he had been told in confidence. But he kept the paper in his wallet, meaning one day to take it to the School of Oriental Studies in London.

He finished his work in Malaya and sailed for home. He had always been a wretched sailor and from the first he was horribly sick and could not leave his bunk. One morning he awoke feeling much better and realized that the ship had mercifully sailed into one of those oases of calm which you may strike in the Indian Ocean, if you are lucky, even in the monsoon. But he wasn't feeling well enough to get up. He lay and gloried in the steadiness of the ship and the absence of those perpetual creak-ings and jarrings and bangings which make a rough passage as hideous to the ear as it is to the stomach. Then he began to be bored and had almost steeled himself into getting out of bed to get a novel from the wardrobe when he remembered the charm in his coat pocket beside his bunk. He could avoid getting up and occupy himself, for the fiftieth time, in trying to make sense out of that rigmarole, in trying to wring from the strange sounds some semblance to any eastern language. Again he failed, and after a while he fell asleep again.

When he awoke he found to his surprise that the ship's surgeon was sitting beside him and watching him with puzzled anxiety.

'You're a fine doctor,' he said. 'For days I've been hoping you would come and either cure me or put me out of my agony, and now, when I'm perfectly well, you come and turn on your damned bedside manner.'

The doctor didn't respond to the jibe. 'I was here all night,' he said, 'and all yesterday and the day before. I thought you were a goner. Does this always happen when you are seasick? If so, for God's sake never leave England again.'

When the doctor had gone Mabbitt found the charm again, screwed up amidst the tangled bedclothes, but he didn't read it again.

'I suppose he must have been right,' he said. 'He seemed an intelligent chap. Hypoglycaemia, he called it. But I had often been seasick before and had never passed out like that. Several times since I've been even worse without passing out. When did you come out here? I had an awful crossing. The Bay was hell. I didn't feel really happy till I saw the old Cecil on the quay at Tangier.'

'But the charm?' I said.

'Oh, the charm. Yes, it's in my safe at the office. I've never taken it to the School of Oriental Studies. After all, how could I tell that the man they put me on to had had his breakfast that morning? Might have had a hangover or something. Often I think I'll get introduced to an orientalist and take him out and give him a damn good lunch and show it to him afterwards, but I'm always too busy for more than a snack at lunch-time, and in the evening there's the train to Purley to catch. But one day I'll do it.'

The silly thing about this story is that I forgot to find out why he was carrying that white rabbit in a brown paper bag.

It was on the way to Marrakech that we passed within sight of the farm of Abdul of the Rats. The story was told me by Jim Wyllie, who was frequently interrupted by the screaming of Moors who, preferring to be clean and hot, wanted the windows shut. Jim, who preferred to be dirty and cool, with still louder screams insisted on opening them. The Moors slowly subsided into a grumbling undertone of opprobrious comment on 'the skull faces' and the story went on.

In those days there was a plague of rats in Morocco and the French engaged rat-catchers, amongst whom was Abdul. A price was placed upon the tail of every rat and Abdul, who was a skilful rat-catcher, prospered exceedingly until one day he remembered that there is no inheritance of acquired characteristics. The rat farm was born and Abdul prospered still more greatly.

The French, accustomed to the unimaginative dishonesty of their own peasantry, were greatly impressed with his skill and would probably have given him the Cross of the Legion of Honour had not rumours reached their ears. The rumours were investigated and Abdul, when next he took to town his batch of rat tails, heard the key turn in the lock behind him. He remained quite calm and admitted everything. With awe-inspiring effrontery he demanded his money. 'There is,' he said, 'nothing in the law as to the origin of the tails.' The French officials, after much poring over official handbooks, admitted that the money must be paid. But, they said, the farm must end. Abdul agreed and demanded a preposterous compensation. The patience of the French wore thin, and Abdul was told roundly that unless he came down to earth and abandoned such ridiculous claims, he would be most illegally shot and the farm destroyed. 'Temper,' said he, 'I beseech you, the cold wind of justice with the warmth of discretion; for unless I return to my farm by midday with the money in my pocket, ten million rats will immediately be released therefrom.'

The money was paid; the rats were slaughtered. Abdul bought some more land and settled down again as a prosperous and law-abiding farmer.

The heavy hand of the Glaui then lay over the whole Atlas. He was more powerful even than the French, whose efforts to curb him were invariably unsuccessful. Although he had a pronounced squint, no woman could resist him. She wisely did not try. In the only possible (albeit almost impossible) hotel, there were staying a young American and his beautiful wife. Her appearance must have been reported accurately to the Glaui, for the couple was invited to a party at the Palace and accepted.

The next day an educated Moor arrived at the hotel and warned them that they must leave at once. If not, he told them, the husband would die. He swept aside the all-powerful American passport as a mere piece of paper. They left.

Another American couple was less lucky. They wished to see the inside of the Mosque in Tangier and would accept no warning. The modern motor cars swept along the street outside, the restaurants were open, the shops were full of modern goods. What could have been safer? They walked into the Mosque and were never seen again.

I was luckier. Separated for a short time from my guide and friend, I stopped a-wandering in Fez and gazed enchanted into the interior of a mosque open to the street. A service was in progress. Suddenly, a Moor seized my arm and exerting all his strength dragged me at a run through a series of complicated alleys. When we stopped, breathless, he explained. 'I heard the crowd round you beginning to murmur. When a crowd here does that, there is going to be trouble. You would have been killed.'

Not only Xauen, but all Morocco was more fun in 1928.

5 Edinburgh Days

I have a very bad memory and the anatomy one was supposed to learn fifty years ago was damnably detailed. One was expected to know everything in Gray's *Anatomy*. I ploughed the examination twice and decided to spend the long vacation sitting at the feet of the famous teacher, Joe Whitaker, of Surgeon's Hall in Edinburgh. I had overspent my allowance, pawned my gold watch, sold the return half of my ticket and acquired a charming dancing partner with whom I spent rapturous hours watching the night sea at Portobello. In short, I was feeling the pinch.

For all its reputation for dour respectability, Edinburgh beneath the surface was a gay city. When a few shillings were available, we would frequent a night club where the available dancing partners were girls of good family, the daughters of distinguished citizens and university professors. I often wondered what story they told their parents.

I shared a bed-sitting-room with John Fulton, later the famous professor of physiology at Yale, even more famous for the collection of old medical books that he presented to the university. At that time he also was feeling the pinch. He initiated me into the sport of book-coping. The rules of this game permit certain deviations from the strictest ethical code; one may not steal, but *caveat emptor*. Often my evening meal and my girl's and our seat in the gallery of the theatre (1s. 6d.) depended on my capacity as a book-coper. I especially remember one evening when the star of the evening was Harry Lauder. He was a small and, at first sight, an insignificant man, dressed in Scottish national dress and always supported by a very crooked walking stick. He achieved in a few minutes a complete hold over his

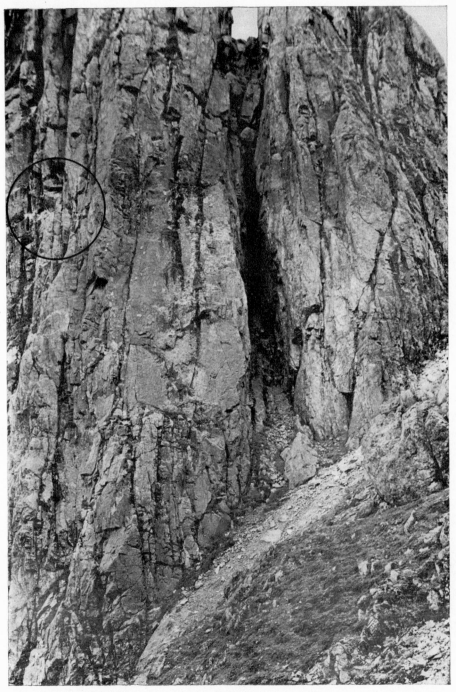

Lead In
The New West Climb on Pillar Rock immediately before the accident

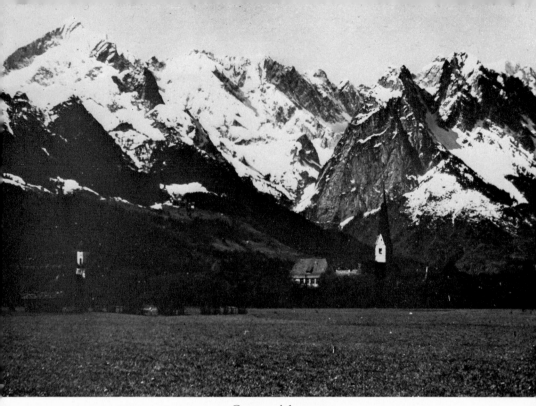

German Adventures
The Wettersteingebirge from Garmisch

German Adventures
The Dreitorspitze

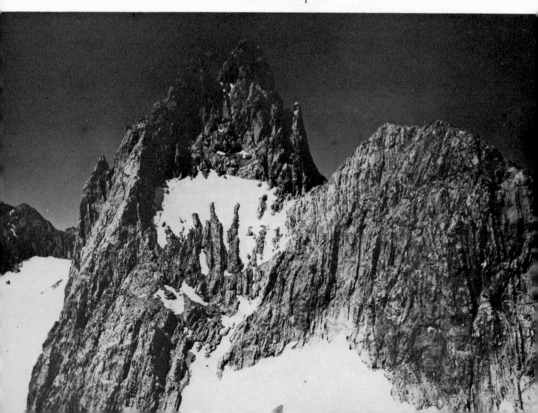

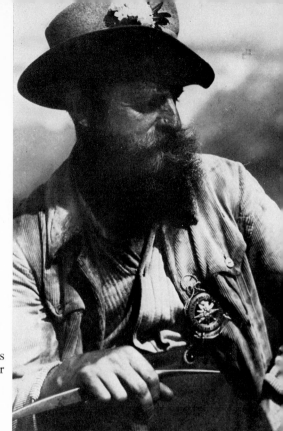

German Adventures
Georg Scheurrer

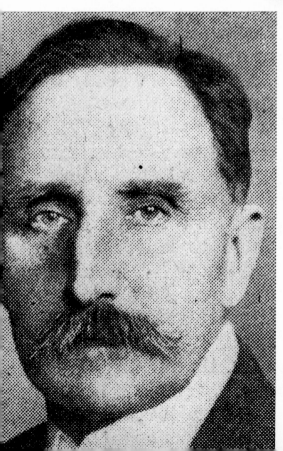

German Adventures
Professor Haushofer

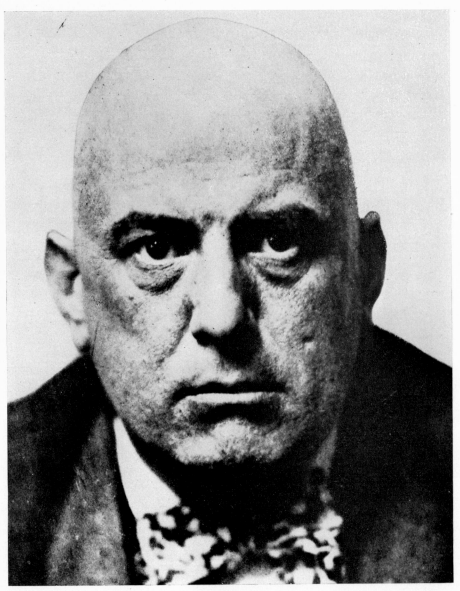

The Beast 666

audience. One night he was the last performer and when he had taken his bow the audience began to leave. Suddenly his voice rang out: 'You have not had the National Anthem. Stand up, you sods! You, there, stop getting into your coat! I'm ashamed that true Scots should behave like that. Stand to attention, damn ye, and sing!' The audience froze to attention and the orchestra began the National Anthem. Not a soul dared to move and the crooked stick conducted them as they sang.

John Grant was never to be deceived; nor would we, even had it been possible, have tried to deceive so trusting a bookseller who would leave one unattended for hours amongst his treasures. However, the rules of the game permitted us to take advantage of his carelessness in sometimes sending, immersed in crates of antique sermons, a minor treasure to the little shop he owned across the road. Later one resold it at a profit of a few welcome shillings to Mr Grant himself at his main shop. Sometimes, too, good things, neglected in odd corners, could be bought during his lunch-time for less than their true value. Once I found the first edition of Coryat's *Crudities* thrown aside as a thing of little value with no price marked within it. I asked the price of the young man at the counter who, remarking that it was nicely bound, suggested ten shillings. Stretching my capital to the utmost, I gave him a note, but he suddenly thought better of it and went to ask his master, unhappily returned unduly early from his lunch. Mr Grant came forth from his office, the treasure held reverently in his hands. 'You want to buy this?' he said. 'Not from you,' I answered, and sadly withdrew.

Mrs Munro had a shop in a by-way off Leith Walk. She had inherited the stock from her father and had two principles on which she priced the books. Every book marked, years before, in her dead father's hand was worth the price he had put on it – no more, no less. All other books were worth half a crown. Thus many books of little value were absurdly dear, while others had become, in a time of changing values, very cheap. Here John Fulton and I found many valuable old medical books which, though priced at far less than their value, were beyond our little means. We had not even enough capital to buy for resale, and knew moreover that one would not have the strength of mind to part with them again. So we hid them in a disused cistern in the back shop to await our return in happier times. A year later, with money in my pocket, I returned to find the house pulled down. By no means could I discover where that cistern had found its last home. I hate to think of a pulped Vesalius interfering with the hygienic arrangements of some surburban villa.

Joe Whitaker was a skinny old man with a straggly white beard, who always wore a white coat with short sleeves that exposed his puny arms. He had a strong objection to note-taking during his lectures. His rule was that we should listen to him with all our ears and in the evening write down all that he had said, word for word. The extraordinary thing was that after a few days we could do it; he was a superb teacher. On our first day he saw a student at the back of the lecture theatre busily taking notes. He ran at surprising speed up the aisle, stretched out a skinny arm, seized the notebook, a large and thick one, tore it horizontally in two and flung it through the window with such force that he broke the glass. Then, without a word, he returned to his lectern and continued the lesson. On one hot August day he noticed one Savage apparently sleeping quietly in the front row.

'Savage, you are asleep.'

'No, sir.'

'Then repeat word for word everything I have said in the last five minutes.'

Savage not only did this but imitated his voice and accent. This time the old man could not at once continue; he was doubled up with laughter.

Every Sunday morning, two or three of us would get up at day-break and repair to Salisbury Crags, just outside the city, where excellent rock climbing could be had. We had to go early in case we should knock down rocks on to strollers on the paths below. Here I nearly ended my climbing days. My friend 'Bunny' Mansell, a novice, was stuck out of my sight above me. Stepping back carelessly to see what had halted him, I fell over the edge of my stance and landed on my back some twenty feet below, happily in a small patch of bog. In doing so, I pulled off 'Bunny' who joined me rather painfully in my bog. Both were unharmed.

We both passed our anatomy examinations. I had decided, should I fail again, to go to the Bar. Thus the country lost, perhaps, a great judge!

Although I dropped the idea of becoming a barrister when I ultimately passed my examination in anatomy, I have never ceased to be fascinated by the courts of law and in my Oxford days I was often called as an expert witness.

The famous Oxford murder was a case in point. The defendant who I have no doubt was guilty, depended in his defence on the exact time at which the murder was committed. The prosecution depended for this on the evidence of Sir Bernard Spilsbury, who as usual was a supremely competent and confident witness. He stated, with all the weight of his enormous reputation, that the death had occurred at just the time at which the defendant could prove no alibi, basing his decision on the exact time at which the tomatoes that the murdered woman had had at her last meal, had reached a particular point in her intestine. I passed a note to the defendant's counsel. 'Is there any evidence about the state of her bowels that day? Had she been constipated? Had she had diarrhoea?' 'Our' Q.C. began his cross-examination in a quiet and respectful way, warmed to his attack, and demanded an opinion from Sir Bernard about these points. Sir Bernard suddenly saw the bits of paper passing between us, looked at me and obviously recognized me as someone whom he had recently examined in forensic medicine. He began to hedge. 'Would I be correct, Sir Bernard,' thundered counsel, 'in suggesting that the evidence you have given is based entirely on your admittedly valuable opinion, rather than a hard-and-fast knowledge of the facts?' 'That,' said Sir Bernard, quietly and obviously shaken, 'is my opinion.' The police surgeon, also called for the prosecution, was almost stone-deaf. A policeman stood beside him and repeated the questions in a shout. The poor man had heard nothing of the previous cross-examination. He merely repeated the opinion he had already heard from the great pathologist.

The judge, who had rather obviously lunched too well, summed up. 'The most eminent forensic scientist of the day has given it as his opinion that death occurred at such and such a time. If you accept this evidence, which I think you must, the defendant's alibi does not stand.'

I lunched afterwards in the Middle Temple when an appeal was discussed. It was decided not to appeal. The defendant was duly hanged. He was probably guilty, but I have often wondered whether sometimes a jury should consider the mental state of a judge, especially after lunch.

No one could put down to a good lunch the biased summing-up of a most learned and respectable judge before whom I later appeared at Winchester Assizes. The trouble with him was a horror of sex.

A young doctor of hitherto unblemished reputation had investigated the case of a teenaged boy whose sexual development was somewhat backward. He had treated him correctly with the pituitary hormone responsible for testicular maturation, but had made the mistake of judging the success of his treatment by the examination of his patient's semen. This involved masturbation at intervals in the surgery. The doctor, according to the evidence, absented himself during this procedure, but a local schoolmaster, said to be in love with the patient and suspicious of what went on, had stationed himself at a window and saw it all. He approached the boy's mother, who remained throughout convinced of the doctor's innocence, and persuaded her to go to the police.

A case was brought before the local magistrate and an eminent physician gave evidence for the prosecution. It was sent to the assizes. The Medical Defence Union asked the senior physician at a famous London hospital and myself to appear for the defence. We interviewed the young doctor and agreed that his motives were innocent.

The prosecution was led by the famous Khaki Roberts, an impressive Rugger international with the reputation of a legal bully. In cross-examination he reduced the unfortunate senior physician to a terrified and stuttering mess, yet his evidence was perfectly sound. It was my turn next. I passed a note to our counsel: 'Please ask me exactly the same questions that you asked my predecessor.' He did, and I repeated word for word what my eminent colleague had said. Khaki's face became darker and darker as the examination proceeded. When it was time for him to cross-examine me he was a deep purple in the face.

'Are you aware, Dr Greene, that you have given the same answers as your predecessor?'

'Yes, sir.'

'Did you hear me say that the last witness was attempting to deceive the court?'

'Yes, sir.'

'Then how have you had the effrontery to give the same answers?'

'Because, sir, they are the only answers that an honest and knowledgeable witness could possibly have given.'

Khaki swept his robe over his shoulder and looking on the point of apoplexy roared in a voice of thunder, 'My Lord, I have finished with this witness.' I returned to my seat and found a note from our counsel: 'Routed, by God.' The jury was convulsed with laughter.

The next witness was the defendant's wife, an exquisite blonde. 'Have you,' said our counsel, 'ever noticed anything abnormal about your husband's sexual behaviour?' 'Oh no, Sir,' she replied, and, blushing prettily, 'on the contrary.' The jury laughed again and the judge sternly admonished them.

He summed up strongly in favour of the prosecution. He had clearly been deeply shocked by so unsavoury a case. He neglected to mention my evidence or that of my distinguished colleague. To his intense disappointment and disgust, the jury found for the defendant without bothering to leave the court. Juries have their uses.

6 General Practice

Sometimes I wonder whether we train our doctors aright. Certainly when I look back on my own student days I am shocked by the amount of rubbish I was taught. Are we teaching rubbish now? I am sure that all I know now about medicine (little though that may be) I have either taught myself or have soaked in by a sort of intellectual osmosis by watching older and wiser men. Perhaps we should go back to the good old days of apprenticeship and dispense with the lectures.

I certainly learned a lot in my first experience of general practice. I was a casualty house surgeon at the old Westminster Hospital in Broad Sanctuary, a lovely neo-Gothic building, admirably suited to be a small hospital. It should have been retained as such when it became necessary for the medical school to expand into the vast complex of buildings near Lambeth Bridge. One of the surgeons asked me whether I would like to take a few weeks leave from the casualty department and join in Wisbech an old Westminster man, Parker by name, whose partners were ill. I went at once.

The night of my arrival was dark, wet and windy, but not as windy as I was. A horse cab took me to the house of the senior partner, Doctor Bullmore, where I was received by his wife and shown immediately to the bedroom of the old man. He was recovering from pneumonia but anxious, before leaving for the South of France, to tell me all I needed to know. 'I'm glad you've come,' he said. 'You will find all the instruments you want in the consulting rooms. Run along now, there's a good fellow. I'm very tired.' A little depressed and frightened, I descended to tea and toast with Mrs Bullmore. I had not gone far with my tea when the door opened and a grey-haired, grey-faced man swayed towards us. 'Are you Greene?' he said. On being reassured on this point he incontinently fainted. My first patient as an independent doctor was thus a colleague with lobar pneumonia, long before 'M. and B.'.

However, Parker was in excellent health and unabashed by his partners' illness. He explained the practice to me. Doctor Bullmore, an F.R.C.S., did general practice, gynaecology and ear, nose and throat surgery. Doctor Butterfield, also F.R.C.S., did general practice, and general surgery. Dr Parker, M.R.C.P., did general practice, pathology and ophthalmology. Each had a beautiful Queen Anne house on the river that flowed through the town, where he did his private practice, and together they shared another beautiful house where they saw their panel patients. This house had a dispensary under a qualified pharmacist, an X-ray plant, and apparatus for physiotherapy. Each partner had a large car and a chauffeur. Each had a holiday of four weeks every year and an additional leave every three years which he spent doing postgraduate study. The three did almost all their own surgery in the local cottage hospital. Should an operation to which they were not accustomed appear to be necessary, the best surgeon in England was summoned to perform it, and his fees paid from partnership funds if the patient could not afford them. The three stood round and watched his every movement. Thereafter if the operation again became advisable they did it themselves.

The efficiency of this group practice, which must have been one of the first in the land, was a thrilling thing for a very young doctor. In my short time in Wisbech, I learned more than in the previous many years of study. It stood me in good stead when I settled in Oxford.

I had qualified and served my turn at Westminster as casualty house surgeon, house physician for children and resident obstetric assistant, with a short term as locum tenens resident medical officer. Donald Paterson, the children's physician, had persuaded Wanders, the manufacturers of baby foods, to endow a registrarship in paediatrics and he offered the post to me. I

45

could not accept. Had I done so my whole life would have been different; I might well have turned wholly to paediatrics and might even have succeeded Paterson. But it was not to be. My father had had to retire because of ill-health and I had to earn my living. In those days registrars were paid £200 per annum. For a long time Dr Counsell of Oxford, with whom I had become intimate in my undergraduate days, had wanted me to join him in general practice, and I decided to go. So began ten years of experience as a general practitioner that I will never regret. I am, I suppose, the only consultant physician in London who has sailed for ten years before the mast.

The Oxford practice was a mixed one. There were the undergraduates who frequented my house in Holywell, the dons whom I usually visited in their colleges, where, too, I often dined, and there were the great houses of the surrounding countryside where I would be given a glass of sherry and a biscuit as I listened to the sorrows of the Lady of the Manor. But the time I most enjoyed was spent in the slums of St Ebbe's and St Thomas's. Such slums no longer exist; they were certainly far worse than anything I had seen when 'on the district' as a student in London. The houses were small, dirty and crowded, the narrow stairs usually hung with filthy, ancient and ragged clothes against which one rubbed as one climbed to the bedroom. They were infested with bugs and I have watched them climbing down the walls as I coped with a difficult delivery a few feet away. Often the roofs leaked whenever it rained and I have seen a steady drip from above on to the bed of an old man with pneumonia. On this occasion, to his astonishment, I tackled a Canon of Christ Church whom I took to task for the state of his college property. 'That,' he said, 'is not my business. You must see the Estates Bursar.' I became very eloquent and quoted the Bible, to him, a Canon! At first he was angry, then puzzled, then distressed. At last he said: 'Young man, you are not I know much of a church-goer, but you have taught me Christianity. Thank you.' The roof was repaired.

But the people who lived in these hovels, now no more, were my main delight in those days. I knew them as I have never been able to know my patients since. Drinking their abominable tea I would listen to their often sordid tales and sometimes I could help. There was the case of the little typist in the family way who sold everything she had except the clothes she stood up in, whose friends in the street gave up without question their few savings, to pay £20 to the abortionist who practised in St Ebbe's as a 'herbalist'. That was my only blackmail. I took £40 off him and we had a grand party in the street that night.

In the same street lived a likeable man, a carpenter, named Gilbert Carter, who unfortunately developed suddenly into a homicidal maniac and had to be 'put away' in the mental hospital at Littlemore. The director there was a skilful and learned man who suffered from excessive optimism concerning the results of his treatment. His patients were often sent home after a short period of residence only to reappear soon, to his chagrin and embarrassment.

So it happened that one day I was summoned urgently to St Ebbe's. The street was completely deserted except for a frightened cluster of women at each end, the men being away at work. Gilbert Carter, apparently in his right mind, received me affably. He was very puzzled by the behaviour of the neighbours and hurt too because of his surly welcome. We sat down to tea in his kitchen while he told me with many expressions of gratitude about his time in Littlemore. The only abnormality I could detect in his behaviour was his insistence on stirring his tea with a carving knife. 'It makes pretty patterns in the tea,' he remarked; 'your spoon ain't nearly so good. I like the look of a knife going round and round in my tea, but it might look even better going round and round in your froat.' So I took the knife away from him and he was very hurt.

A lot of my Oxford patients seemed to be a little mad, whether they belonged to the town or the gown. There was, for instance, Alice Drake. She was a very talented old lady, a musician and a dramatist of distinction. She had never married and the reason was too clear. Tall, gaunt, rather masculine of physique, her lined face had been terribly scarred by an unwise physician who in her youth had attempted to cure its excessive hairiness with a course of X-ray treatment. The hair had gone, true, but in its place was red and puckered skin. Those who have seen the terrible faces of airmen burned in Hitler's war may guess at her appearance.

But she showed no sign of being conscious of this. Sensible, matter-of-fact, full of interest in the world about her, her conversation had such charm that after a little one forgot her ravaged face. So when she came to me with her story one could hardly disbelieve her.

She was, she said, in danger of death at the hands of the Professor of Music whom she had crossed over some matter of administration in the world of music in the University. He was determined to have his way and could only achieve it by her death. He would follow her through the streets, hoping that she would take some by-way in which he could club her to death unobserved. She dared not take any unfrequented road. Once in Hell Passage, that narrow dark lane that runs between Holywell and New College Lane, passing right through the Turf Tavern, she had heard his footsteps behind her and, teetotaller though she was, had been forced to take refuge in the bar and ask a kindly undergraduate to escort her to her home. Then he had turned to subtler methods. She had seen him in her grocer's shop in quiet converse with one of the assistants, and had seen money pass and had had to buy her food elsewhere. In every food shop she frequented she had seen the incident repeated. Again his method changed. She was in the habit of taking her lunch in a little café in St Clement's. He too began to lunch there and to try to join her at her table and to feign distress when she refused his company. He always carried with him a little glass tube that he said contained saccharine, but she knew that it was a deadly poison that would be slipped into her coffee if her attention wandered for a moment. After a while he ceased his importunity, but every day without fail she would see his face, peering through the window of the café, thinking of some new way of destroying her.

She came to see me often, always with a new story of the Professor's malignancy, always told in a calm voice with no hint of hysteria. Had I not known the Professor as a kindly man who would not hurt a fly I might have been deceived. She was most plausible. I could never make her see that her imagination was playing tricks with her; had I been older and more experienced I would not have tried. The manner of her recitation was such that even I, convinced of her insanity whenever we were apart, had momentary doubts. When she told me of his face at the café window I saw my chance of proving her wrong. I arranged to have lunch with her there. As the meal progressed she became worried at his failure to appear and I began to push home my point.

Suddenly the worry left her face and fear took its place. She stared towards the window and I swung round expecting an innocent stranger. Pressed hard against the glass, the eyes searching the room, was the unmistakable face of the Professor of Music.

Mrs Bidwell was a tall, austere, bespectacled woman in her thirties, who came from Cardiff. She talked nonsense about her symptoms with the air of an expert educating a moron. Her symptoms were varied, frequent and bizarre.

One day her sister telephoned to say that she had a bad discharge from an abdominal scar, said to be the result of an appendicectomy three years before. When I saw her I found no discharge, but in the middle of the scar was an area that, when seen through a magnifying glass, was obviously self-inflicted with a razor blade. In those days I rather fancied myself as a psychiatrist, so I tried to get her to admit the truth. Failing by ordinary conversational means, I hypnotized her. She readily admitted the truth and told me a long and sad story about her miserable life with a brutal husband. She had made the wound on her abdomen in the hope that she would be sent to hospital. I released her from her trance and she left somewhat comforted.

The next morning her sister telephoned and asked me whether Mrs Bidwell was still with me. Annoyed by this insult to my good taste, I replied indignantly that she was not. 'Well,' said her sister, 'she hasn't been home since she left to see you.' I told her to tell the police. A few minutes later, a ward sister telephoned from the Radcliffe Infirmary to say that Mrs Bidwell had been brought in the night before suffering from loss of memory but seemed to be all right again. Could she be discharged? I told the sister that it was most improper for her to ask such a question of a general practitioner and that she must ask the permission of the consultant in charge of her case. Later her husband telephoned to say that he had fetched her home; he sounded a mild and rather effeminate person. He told me that she was 'going convalescent' to her father. Her father then telephoned to learn all the details. I was getting rather tired of Mrs Bidwell, but my conscience was not quite clear and I remained in consequence reasonably polite, and the telephone continued to ring. A nurse rang from the Radcliffe to tell me she had left. The police-woman rang to tell me the same thing. A chemist's assistant rang to ask whether he could repeat her medicine; curious that, for it was only a harmless mixture for indigestion and needed no prescription.

It was when Mrs Bidwell telephoned to say 'goodbye' and to thank me for all my kindness that it occurred to me that it was a curious coincidence that Mrs Bidwell, her sister, her husband, her father, a sister and a nurse at the hospital, a policewoman and a chemist's assistant all had slight Welsh accents and sounded a trifle effeminate. 'Mrs Bidwell,' I said, 'I'm tired of your telephone calls and it must be very expensive for you.' The scream of indignation she emitted startled the pigeons in my garden.

I still feel sad about one of my Oxford patients, a dear old lady whose most treasured possession was her tom-cat. He followed her like a dog and obviously returned the affection she lavished on him. One early morning she telephoned in great distress; Tom had gone mad and had attacked her as she slept. He had scratched her and bitten her round her waist. I went at once and found that she had shingles. I joyfully assured her that she had had a nightmare and that Tom was innocent. 'Where is he?' I asked. 'I will bring him to you and you can apologize.'

To my surprise, far from welcoming the glad news, she burst into bitter tears. Before I came she had sent for the vet and had had Tom destroyed.

Giveen of Wadham undoubtedly had a hole in his mind. I realized this very soon, when climbing with him; he was completely without physical fear. I don't mean merely that he was very brave: to suggest this would be tantamount to saying that a man who is not hungry should be praised for not eating. He just didn't need to be brave.

The ascent of the Martyrs' Memorial had become unpopular in my undergraduate days because the Oxford University Mountaineering Club believed, like all reputable climbing clubs, in a reasonable respect for human life, especially one's own: the 'rock' of which the Memorial was built was very friable. Giveen, when he climbed it, did a lot of damage, but felt sufficiently secure to leave a chamber-pot on the summit. This had been done before, reputedly on the last occasion, by Leo Amery, later to be President of the Alpine Club and First Lord of the Admiralty. Giveen was the first to wire it on, so that it could not, as on previous occasions, be removed with a hose by the fire-brigade. A scaffold had to be erected at great expense. I think that it was on this occasion that someone asked the Professor of Ornithology whether it was a fact that a nightjar had recently built a nest on the summit of the Martyrs' Memorial. The culprit was suspected by the proctors, but there was no real evidence against him and no action could be taken in the face of his bland denials. His appearance was always in his favour – small, fair-haired and pink and white, he resembled the *putti* of mediaeval Italian paintings. Perhaps he came nearer to justice on an occasion on which he was utterly innocent. He was accused by his landlady of committing the intolerable nuisance of having what she described as 'pinted ores' in his room. 'And me, I 'as to wash em.' It was only after a long judicial inquiry that it was established that the 'ores' were oars and not whores. Eventually I believe he was sent down, for what offence I have now forgotten.

Before his departure he sold me his car, a small 10-horsepower Talbot. I had paid for it and had it for a few days when it disappeared. He had told me that all necessary tools were in the boot. On examination the boot was found to contain a corkscrew, a bottle opener and a generous supply of contraceptives. Soon afterwards I saw Giveen driving it up the Cornmarket and caught him in a traffic block. He wasn't at all embarrassed. 'You see,' he said, 'my father gave it to me and objects to my selling it.' 'All right,' I said, 'but what about the money?' 'I will send you a cheque today,' he said. He did and it bounced. I telephoned to him at his home and was answered by his father, an eminent barrister, who wormed the truth out of me. 'I had no objection,' he said, 'to his selling the car. I shall send you a refund at once, and I would warn you never again to have any financial dealings with my son'; it must have been a hard thing for a father to say to a stranger.

Giveen was proposed for membership of the Climbers' Club. When his name came up before the Committee, of which I was a member, I black-balled him. Somebody told him and I had a very hurt letter from him, written more in sorrow than in anger. Soon after I was in the climbers' hut at Helyg in the Ogwen Valley and was being attacked by a kind man for excluding such a fine climber from the club. In the middle of the discussion Giveen walked in and greeted me effusively as an old friend. His charm soon thawed the ice, and he and the friends who had brought him, Stott, Taylor and one I will call T. in case he is still alive, were the life and soul of the party.

Next day I had to return home. T., Taylor and Stott were novices in the mountains, but that did not deter Giveen from taking them up one of the longest and stiffest climbs in North Wales, the great gully of Craig-yr-Ysfa. It was a wet day, when the rocks in all gully climbs are unpleasantly greasy. The party was probably tired and wet when it reached the foot of the climb, two hours of rough walking from the hut, and the inexperience of three of the four, especially in such conditions, delayed them so much that it was already dark when they reached the top. They must have been played out, cold, miserable, tired, hungry. With only one lantern to guide them they began what in daylight was the easy way home, but which in such conditions was terrible. They dropped their compass and couldn't find it; the lantern expired. At 8 p.m. Taylor fell into a tarn and Stott, in utter darkness, dived in, found him and dragged him to the shore, where he collapsed. Giveen said that he dragged Taylor and Stott to the shelter of a rock and descended with T., 'as rapidly as possible' to Helyg, which they reached at 2.15 a.m. where they had a rapid snack and 'drove as rapidly as possible to the hotel at Pen-y-gwryd' for help, arriving at 6.20 a.m. A rescue party set out and found the dead bodies of Taylor and Stott. It is a 20-minute drive from Helyg to Pen-y-gwryd. It seems certain that between 2.25 and 6.00 a.m. they slept happily.

But Stott's father was not satisfied by Giveen's evidence at the inquest. Another party set out. They found Taylor's watch beside the tarn; it had stopped at 6.40. What had happened in those twelve hours?

It soon became clear that Giveen and T. had abandoned the other two, still alive, in the early evening, had reached Helyg and had there had a good meal and gone to bed. Only the next morning did they go to Pen-y-gwryd for help. The two other men, without the extra clothing the survivors could have given them, had tried to struggle on and had collapsed in a few inches of water and there had drowned. The inquest was not reopened, but the story was soon known to all in the climbing fraternity. Giveen 'got away with it' but from then on nourished an obsessional hatred against me, who had blocked his entry to the Climbers' Club.

I forget how long afterwards came the sequel. I lived then in Holywell, a long old street in Oxford where many doctors lived. Maurice Bowra, the Warden of Giveen's former college, telephoned to me and told me that the Chief Constable had told him that Giveen was in Oxford (illegally, as he had been 'sent down') and had said in a local pub that he was there to 'get' me. I didn't take this at all seriously, but a few nights later he followed someone, a tall man like me, down Holywell and out of the city to the wild open space of Port Meadow. There he shot the man, a complete stranger, in the back, happily not fatally, and turned the other barrel on himself, this time fatally. Perhaps it was all for the best.

I have met many men unfit to be parents but none as unfit as O'Shanter senior. He bullied little Tam unmercifully through his childhood, trying to turn a small and sensitive boy into the tough he felt his son should be. At Oxford Tam might have found some refuge but his father, who gave him a ludicrously small allowance, made a habit of descending upon him unannounced and chiding him for his extravagance. It is hardly surprising that Tam developed thyrotoxicosis. His father refused at first to pay Sir Thomas Dunhill's fee for the operation that he had to undergo on the grounds that he had never heard of any such disease, but Sir Thomas too could be tough. Not long afterwards I found that Tam had pulmonary tuberculosis. The father had it fixed in his mind that this was a disease due to neglect and malnutrition. Moreover he had heard of it. I seized my chance, underlined his erroneous views and put the blame squarely on his shoulders. He broke down, wept and performed a complete volte face, but it was too late to retain Tam's affection.

Amidst these complications of life, it is hardly surprising that Tam took to drink. I struggled with him for a whole term and finally told him the brutal truth. 'Tam' I told him, 'if you don't go completely on the wagon you will be dead in five years.'

By then we were friends and it was six o'clock. Suddenly the consulting-room ceased to be and became my library. My patient ceased to be and became my friend. The doctor in me ceased to be, remembering only that a stressful hour had ended. 'Well,' I said. 'That's that. Let's have a drink.' We realized simultaneously what I had said and the laughter that followed solved the problem. For the first time Tam refused a drink.

The years went by and I kept in touch. He remained a teetoller and became a successful journalist. One night we were dining at the Athenaeum and in the drawing-room later he saw my hand go out to the drink that wasn't there. 'Raymond,' he said. 'I have lost all urge to drink. But somehow a drink at the end of a good evening seems right and proper and obviously you would like one. Do you think I could risk it? If you say "no", I won't.' I said 'yes'.

So there we sat, sipping our brandies, till suddenly I saw Tam's startled gaze fixed over my left shoulder. He pushed away his glass and let his head sink on his anguished hands. Turning, I saw six bishops, all clad in purple, standing in line, each with a whisky in his hand. It was the evening of the Lord Mayor's banquet to the bishops, most of whom were members of the Club. Tam soon recovered but he never took the risk again.

Everybody liked Denzil Batchelor. He had a persistently hypomanic personality, even when he was sober, a relatively rare condition. When he was drunk, he exuded buoyancy and charm; to him, everything was funny. He hardly ever stopped laughing and it was impossible not to laugh with him. So when his father suggested that he should live with me in Holywell and be cured of his addiction, I gladly agreed.

There was another reason; I was desperately in debt. I had borrowed all I could to buy a half-share in a prosperous practice. Within a few weeks of my arrival, before he had had a chance of introducing me to his private patients, Counsell went into the Oxford Eye Hospital with glaucoma and remained there for many months. The private practice melted rapidly away; the panel remained, but I had paid in effect twice as much as the practice was worth. When he returned, his sight was very bad and it gradually deteriorated, though how much I did not realize until a long time after he was completely blind. He was a superb actor, and so lovable a man that one didn't want to know. Meanwhile my task was gradually to build up the private practice again. Ultimately I succeeded, but in 1930 my position was still insecure. I was glad to accept the job of curing Denzil of his 'alcoholism'.

In fact he was not an alcoholic at all. He gave up drinking quickly and with a good grace. I think I suffered more; I like my drink but never drank in Denzil's presence. He got a job as a reporter on the *Oxford Mail* when my friend Charles Fenby was editor, but he wasn't much good. One evening he came back to Holywell in an unusual state of depression. Charles had put him on the mat. 'Denzil,' he had said. 'You are no good as a reporter. You always arrive too late. The good reporter gets there first, even before anything has happened.'

Denzil and I were both hard up, but we had a friend, Giles Playfair, who was in even lower water. In his case something had got to be done about it and done quickly. He conceived the Oxford University Balloon Union. In the *Isis*, of which he was editor, he advertised the forthcoming revival in the home of lost causes of the ancient and honourable sport of ballooning. For the princely sum of one shilling one could become an original member. Giles had some important friends in the London journalistic world and the great news spread. Tallulah Bankhead wrote an article on ballooning in the *Evening Standard*, which tactfully did not inquire whether she had ever ballooned. The money flowed in and Giles was in the black again.

However, a few tactless original members began to ask when the balloon would go up. Something had to be done about it. Giles borrowed the grounds of the Oxford Gas Works, hired a balloon and a balloonist, and organized with admirable efficiency the opening meet of the Club. Denzil meanwhile had seen his Great Opportunity to prove Charles Fenby wrong. Not only had he learned from Giles the details of the meet; he was going up in the balloon. I was the Honorary Medical Officer (non-playing).

The great event was preceded by a lunch party with Sir Nigel, Giles's father, in the chair. I still have the menu, signed by my table companions, Giles Playfair, Glen Byam Shaw, Anthony Mathias, one whose signature I cannot read and – Tallulah Bankhead. It was an ornate production, and included a magnificent unsigned poem glorifying the balloon. We ate Huîtres Montgolfier, Dindon à la Ballonier, Salade Gordon Bennett, Orange Glace Gambetta and Café au Brewer. The wines are not mentioned but I remember that they were plentiful and good. At intervals telegrams arrived from very important people, including the Secretary of State for Air, who welcomed the spirit of the University in reviving so noble a sport. Speeches followed, and then the company left for the Gas Works.

Here the great balloon lay ready in the expert hands of its skipper. Giles, Denzil and one Hugh Speaight, clad in fur coats and deer-stalker caps, boarded the craft. Near by stood the lovely Tallulah, holding by a piece of string a miniature balloon. Precisely on time she cut the string with golden scissors and the little balloon sailed upwards into the cloudless sky. The big one remained *in situ*. The aeronauts jettisoned their fur coats; a noble gesture. Amidst the plaudits of the vast throng (each member of which had paid a shilling at the gate), Tallulah was given another toy balloon and another piece of string. Once more the golden scissors snipped and the little balloon followed its predecessor into the empyrean. Once more the big balloon stayed put, and the crowd began to laugh. Then they jettisoned Denzil. The third time was lucky.

Denzil, for once deeply depressed, Hugh's brother Robert, desperately anxious, and Tallulah, vastly amused, piled into my small car and tried to follow the balloon across the Oxfordshire countryside. Soon we lost it. Once we caught up with the lorry that was supposed to meet it on its descent, but the lorry too had lost its way, so we sat in the back and drank bottled beer, and decided to return to Oxford.

When we came to my house, we heard a voice in my consulting-room. Hugh Speaight was at my telephone dictating an account of the flight to an evening paper. As we entered the room we heard his last sentence. 'Amongst those who were present to welcome the balloon as it landed was Mr Charles Fenby, the editor of the *Oxford Mail*.'

Denzil gave a wild and piercing scream and left immediately for Australia.

I used often to drive between Oxford and London. There were three possible routes, by Iffley and Henley; by Cowley and High Wycombe; and by Thame and Aylesbury. Even in the twenties the first two routes were reasonably good but the last, at any rate between Thame and Aylesbury, was little more than a lane. There were frequent unexpected bends and sometimes the straight road ahead was the wrong one. On a fine summer day the route had its advantages; it was more beautiful and more rural and wild flowers grew in the high hedges and the birds sang. Small animals, anxious for an unexplained reason to reach the other side, would make one's journey slow, but to choose it on a stormy winter night was very silly, and as I drove along, I tried unsuccessfully to remember why I had done it. I must, I thought, have had my mind on some problem, but I couldn't think of any problem. If I had been absent-minded I would surely have taken my usual route up the Iffley Road, especially as my small and ancient Morris Cowley didn't really enjoy the steepness of Headington Hill.

The rain teemed down from a starless moonless sky into a darkness that could be felt, and my headlights were too weak to do more than reflect on to my windscreen, cleared only intermittently by an inefficient manually operated wiper, the small confusing facets of falling water.

At first I knew my way, but soon I was off my own ground. Slowing to peer through the driving rain at a signpost designed to be invisible by any traveller not mounted on a horse of at least sixteen hands, I discovered a curious and alarming fact. The brilliance of my headlights was in direct relationship with the speed of my car. If I drove fast, I could see moderately well some twenty yards ahead. If, my natural caution awakened by a narrow twisting lane, I slowed to a safe speed, the headlights became dim enough to undo any beneficial effects of my caution. If I stopped altogether to examine a signpost, they went out altogether and I had to restart the car in absolute darkness which persisted until I was well under way – or had hit a bank, in which case it settled on me again like a pall. After several such incidents, a straight bit of lane gave me an opportunity to see again and I determined to keep going and to risk no more signposts. By this time I was entirely lost, but I was not much worried by the thought because I felt sure that eventually my lane must run into a road and the road into a well-lit town, where, even if I could not find a garage, I could at least take my bearings and strike a main road to London along which I could go at a speed great enough to keep my lights in being. Instead, the lanes grew narrower and more muddy, and I ran between hedges higher and more unkempt. It became steadily more hazardous to keep up the twenty-five miles an hour, short of which the darkness descended on me again. And then, straight across my path, uncompromisingly obstructive, there appeared a gate.

I stopped and utter darkness, the darkness of the pit, descended. I could, of course, feel my way to the gate and open it. I might even be able to overcome in time the natural and improper tendency of farm gates to close themselves as soon as one had regained one's car. But what lay beyond? Into what field or farm yard or gravel pit or quarry would I drive in utter darkness until the speed of twenty-five miles an hour had been attained again?

On the other hand, far off, across I could not tell how many fields, I saw a lonely light. Capitulation was obviously the wisest course. I abandoned ship and set off towards that hope of salvation – an improbable hope, for I was in the depths of the countryside and it was by now long past midnight. As I forced my way through hedges and floundered through ditches, I became aware of the fact that I had dined early and that I was very hungry. For food I could hardly hope, but some straw to sleep on was by this time an attractive prospect.

I fell into another ditch, climbed a crumbling ha-ha, ruined a bed of daffodils and found my farm.

The apologetic sound of my knock was followed at once by the shambling of unsteady feet, and the largest man I have ever seen stood in the lighted doorway. Legs like oaks supported a massive torso, beside which hung great arms as long and as hairy as a gorilla's, and high in the shadow above the lantern in the porch a great moon-like face framed in grey hair peered out into the darkness. Stories of motiveless murders in dark haunted farms rushed back to me before I had time to realize that the giant was very friendly, and very drunk. He dragged me within as though he was expecting me, and into his dining-room where the table was laid for two. We had an excellent dinner. Why had he not already dined? I asked. He didn't remember. Who was he expecting? He didn't remember. When we had eaten, almost in silence, he showed me to a room, neat and clean and obviously ready for a guest. There was no one else in the house.

With some difficulty, I found my car in the darkness, and carried my suitcase back to the house. The old man was at the whisky bottle again, and I joined him. We sat almost in silence till he rose and moved, swaying heavily, through the door. There was a loud crash, and rushing through to the next room, I found he had fallen over the electric fire and was lying unconscious on the floor with his clothes already well alight. I easily extinguished the flame before it touched his body, turned him into 'the coma position', put a cushion under his head, and went to bed and to sleep.

In the morning he was sleeping quietly and I thought it best to leave him. I wrote a note of thanks and left. There was no difficulty in finding the car then. On that bright morning the headlights blazed across the intervening fields. They never gave any trouble again.

Three questions I have often asked myself. Why did I take that road? What went wrong with my headlights? For whom was dinner waiting and a bed prepared?

Anderson was a very distinguished lepidopterist. He would probably have been a professor but for one failing; he was hardly ever sober. As the years went by he needed more and more alcohol to assist him to the state of bliss. He was staying at the King's Arms Hotel at the junction of the Broad and Holywell when the D.T.'s got him. He locked himself in his room and demanded to be supplied with whisky by a string let down from his window. The landlady at first complied, then sent for me. He knew me well and I thought that we were friends. After a long colloquy he decided to open the door and I found myself faced with a revolver, whether loaded or not I did not then know. I decided to ignore it. He kept me covered while he told me the story. The walls of his room were, he said, completely covered with butterflies, but they differed from most of their genus in being supplied with stings. They seemed to be worried by his revolver and he had been able to keep them at bay just by waving it at them. He didn't want to kill them for they were beautiful specimens. Then suddenly he fired. The bullet went past my right ear and hit the brass knob of the door with a loud crash. 'I'm so sorry,' he said, 'but that one was obviously coming for me. What a pity; as a specimen he's ruined.'

The trouble was that the Vice-Chancellor and the Chief Constable were in league against him. He could not go out because the hotel was surrounded. 'That,' I said, 'is where I can help. The Chief Constable is an old friend of mine. He has one unfortunate failing – he drinks too much. If I can lure him into my partner's house, only a few doors away, we can soon get him into a condition in which he will do anything I tell him. The watchers round the hotel are all police – no bulldogs. I will persuade him to call them off and can then smuggle you out to a country house owned by a friend of mine a few miles outside the city. By the time he comes round you will be gone. You can lie low there until the hue and cry has subsided.'

This seemed to him to be a good idea. I went to Dr Counsell's house and telephoned to the Warneford Mental Hospital. The superintendent was with difficulty persuaded from sending an ambulance and some attendants. I told him that Anderson was a crack shot, that he wouldn't give up his gun and that his plan would mean bloodshed. I said I would bring him in my car. I gave enough time for the fictitious Chief Constable to drink a fictitious bottle of whisky and returned to the hotel, the inhabitants of which had prudently left. Anderson was most grateful, but he would not give up his gun and I did not want to make him suspicious by insisting. We crept like two conspirators to my car and were about to leave when he suddenly applied the hand-brake. 'Now, what's the trouble?' I said. 'We must be quick. The Chief Constable may sober up at any moment and put the watchers on again.' 'I think,' he said, 'there is just time for me to shoot the landlady, who must have been in the conspiracy.' 'Look out,' I cried, 'don't you see the constable in that shadow?' He fired into the empty shadow, I took off the brake and we were away.

I wondered what would happen when the high stone wall of the Warneford loomed above us, and began to prepare the ground. I explained that my friend was a recluse who also had been persecuted by the Vice-Chancellor, the Chief Constable and the landlady of the King's Arms, who was, of course, their mistress. In consequence he had built an impregnable wall round his property. This, Anderson said, was a very wise pre-caution. The great gates swung open as we approached and I knew that the most dangerous moment had come, but Anderson, who had been sitting tautly beside me with his gun on his knee, suddenly relaxed. 'I feel safe here,' he said. 'Will you do some-thing for me? I would like you to kill that landlady.' 'Certainly,' I replied, 'but I haven't a gun.' 'Then take mine,' he said. 'I shan't need it here.'

7 Cloak without Dagger

I suppose that there is a romantic child, or a Walter Mitty, in most grown men, usually suppressed but occasionally breaking surface. Why otherwise should books about spies sell so well? Why should such men as Philby, traitors though they may be, appeal to the imagination of so many of us?

I first found this flaw in myself in the highly unlikely circumstances of the high table at the little Oxford college of St Edmund Hall. I was dining there one evening before my Kamet adventure. Someone who knew my plans asked me for more details. Someone I did not know showed a flattering interest, asked me many relevant questions, asked me in particular how I proposed to come back from the Zaskar range. I said that I was planning to return conventionally on a P. & O. ship from Bombay. He asked me whether I had thought of returning by land through Afghanistan and Russia. The idea appealed to me but, not having thought of it before, I expressed only a slight interest in the suggestion. No more was said. It was years later that I identified my questioner; he became General Sir Bernard Paget, but was then unknown to fame.

A week passed before I found on my breakfast table a buff envelope addressed to Lieut. C. R. Greene, R.A.M.C. (T.A.). It contained a polite request that at my earliest convenience I would call on General Templeton at the War Office. I went.

General Templeton received me courteously and explained that he proposed to send me on to Colonel Murray, into whose presence I was immediately shown.

'I gather,' he said, 'that you are going on the Kamet expedition

63

and that you might be persuaded to return by way of Afghanistan and Russia?' I hesitated a little, but admitted that the idea had been put into my head.

'We would like to send someone who has had some military training, and who is also a mountaineer. We want to know how easy it would be for the Russians to invade India by way of Afghanistan. We want more information about the possible routes by Merv or Mazar-i-Sharif. Could they come over in strength, or, as some have said, would they have to trickle over and concentrate, here or here (he pointed to a large map on the wall) before progressing in force.'

'But surely,' I said, 'you have your own men there to tell you?'

'Curiously enough,' he replied, 'we have men there with some military knowledge, but none who are mountaineers. That is where you could help.'

Of course, being only thirty, I was excited and immediately agreed. We spent the morning poring over the map.

'You will, of course, arrange my journey?'

'No. You must go as an ordinary tourist. We might later be able to arrange an ex-gratia payment, but you must go on your own. You must arrange your journey with the India Office and with the Russians without mentioning us. This should be easy.'

I went across to the India Office and was received by a pleasant person who without hesitation turned down the project.

'You would probably run into trouble and we would have to get you out.'

'But supposing I were to say, in writing if you like, that I would not ask for your help?'

'No good; it would still be our duty, whatever you had said.'

The conversation continued in a most friendly way. Suddenly he said: 'Surely we have met before: Oxford, perhaps?'

'I thought your face was familiar.'

'Did you know Tommy Creed?'

'Yes, he was one of my best friends in Oxford days, but since he went to the Sudan I have not seen him.'

'Do you remember a night in his rooms in the Broad, when he persuaded P.C. 51 to come up from his beat and drink with us?'

'Of course, I remember the time well.'

We continued to exchange reminiscences of Oxford. Suddenly he looked at the clock.

'I'm sorry, but I am late for another appointment. About this journey; I think it can be arranged. When do you want to go?'

The Russians were even easier. There was no objection except that the recommendation would have to go to Moscow, where they might be very slow in issuing the necessary papers. By the time they came I would have left. So I arranged for the permission to be sent to me at Simla, for me to collect on my return from Kamet. Meanwhile, with the aid of a map given me by Colonel Murray, I planned my journey northwards to Mazar-i-Sharif through the Hindu Kush, and then westwards to Merv.

The end of the story is an anticlimax. Kamet over, I arrived in Simla where a letter from Moscow awaited me. Permission was emphatically refused. I cabled to the War Office and my instructions were definite: 'On no account go.' The only lesson to be learned from this banal incident is that even Oxford Senior Common Rooms may be 'bugged'. I still have my map.

It was a disappointment to the Walter Mitty within me, and I did not again establish my connection with the Old Firm for ten years, when I found myself involved with the Combined Operations Executive and the Special Operations Executive in Hitler's war. Apparently, I had already been 'cleared'.

Naturally, as a doctor with the Kamet Expedition and the Everest Expedition of 1933, I had made a special study of mountain medicine and, in particular, of rescue operations. While Sir Roger Keyes was still the Chief of Combined Operations, I was often summoned to Richmond Terrace and asked my advice about the transport of wounded away from the hazardous attacks the Commandos made on the coast of Europe. Sir Roger seemed to the officers I met unduly cautious, and the change in morale when he was succeeded by Lord Louis Mountbatten was like a shaft of light into a darkened room. Everyone was at once on his toes. My main task was to design a means of getting away not only the wounded but also the dead. The Germans were, it was said, extremely shaken if, when the raid was over, there were no dead enemies to be found. I evolved what came to be known as the Greene Carrier, which was based on the Bergen frame; a sort of rucksack without a bag, by means of which a single man could carry away a dead or unconscious comrade without assistance. I don't think it was much used by the Commandos but proved very useful in the Burma campaign, as a result of which, I received the generous 'award to inventors' of £300, on which sum I had to pay income tax.

On the orders of Lord Louis, I returned to rock-climbing, of which I had done little since my marriage seven years earlier. I was ordered to train the Commando medical officers in the art of getting wounded down cliff faces. Obviously they had first to be taught the techniques of rock-climbing, and I had several happy climbing holidays in North Wales, a pleasant change from teaching students the whole of medicine, from dermatology to neurology, at Aylesbury. I had another pleasant holiday inspecting the various Commandos training on the west coast of Scotland, to ensure that their use of the Greene Carrier was well-understood. Of this holiday I particularly remember the difficulty I had in extracting my expenses from the financial secretary of the War Office. After several months of useless and time-wasting correspondence, I had a letter that laid the whole blame on me. I had, it appears, claimed ten shillings less than was probably owing to me, and I had wasted a lot of valuable time of the clerical staff in determining which sum was correct, a problem on which it was still working. I replied that I didn't mind a b—— which amount was paid me, and added that the inefficiency of his department was such that I was surprised that we had not yet lost the war. The money came by return of post; the larger sum.

A little straight talk to officials is often effective. Some years earlier, when I was the regimental medical officer of the Fourth Battalion of the Oxfordshire and Buckinghamshire Light Infantry, my sergeant reported that at the annual audit it had been found that one sewing machine needle was missing. This, he said, must be reported.

'All right, so what?'

'It means a court of inquiry, sir.'

'What does this involve?'

'A medical officer from the Division, sir, and a gentleman from the War Office. They will stay at the Randolph Hotel and look over all our stores and find out who is to blame.'

After a number of letters had passed between the battalion, the division and the War Office, it was decided that an inquiry should be held. I wrote a final letter which read: 'Cost of inquiry to tax-payer, probably £10. Value of needle, 6d. Please find attached one 6d. stamp, and for God's sake don't go on being so bloody silly.' I heard no more.

It was while I was with the Fourth Oxford and Bucks Light Infantry that I clashed again with authority. I went for annual training to a camp in the Isle of Wight, where I found myself the senior medical officer. The camp, which contained not only some hundreds of men, but also a large number of horses, was supplied with water by a pipe one half of an inch in diameter. A little simple arithmetic showed that it could not supply enough water unless it flowed continuously, but as demands were not continuous much of it would be wasted. The answer was obvious; we must have storage tanks to accumulate water at times of lesser demand. I found the contractor, who, with speed and efficiency, erected two enormous tanks into which the little pipe continuously discharged its meagre flow.

The next day the Brigadier, known as Tim, whose responsibility it had been to set up the camp, arrived in a very bad temper. He gave an infuriated look at the tanks, slapped his boots and demanded to see the contractor, from whom he demanded an explanation. The contractor replied, 'Orders of the Medical Officer, sir.' He turned on me in fury. I gave my explanation in simple terms. He swallowed his anger and continued his inspection.

Meanwhile, I had, as part of my normal duty, inspected the latrines. These consisted of trenches dug in the field above the

Moments of Being

camp, which lay on a rather steep slope below them. The soil was only a few inches deep and the subsoil was impermeable clay; in consequence there was a continuous seepage of sewage down the hill, through the tents and, more important still, through the cook-house. I had therefore given orders for deep pits to be dug between the latrines and the tents, calculating that they were large enough to contain the sewage during our two weeks there. The pits were covered with large pieces of corrugated iron, on the edge of one of which the Brigadier unfortunately tripped. Turning to the pioneer sergeant, he shouted, 'What is this junk doing here? Can't you keep the place tidy? Take it away.' The sergeant explained that they covered cesspits. The Brigadier turned on me a purple face. 'You again?' he shouted. 'Yes, sir.' I replied quietly and enlightened him about my reasons. He was beginning to weaken. 'So I suppose this is my fault too?' 'Yes, sir.' 'How the Hell could I tell?' 'If, sir, you would be kind enough to walk with me about fifty yards to the edge of the cliff you will be able to see the stratification of the hill.' He came with me and spoke no more. I had free drinks in the mess that day.

During my time with Combined Operations I had a most enjoyable trip to Scapa Flow, the object of which was partly to entertain the troops with my Himalayan experiences and partly to warn them about the dangers of frostbite, trench foot and immersion foot. I had always been a bad sailor. Starting in a drifter out towards a guard-ship in the Atlantic, I wedged myself beside the skipper with a bucket between my knees and instructed him to take no notice of me. After a while he looked round at me and, slightly aggrieved, said, 'You are not being sick.' 'It must,' I replied, 'be your enthralling conversation.' But it wasn't. I lectured in the hold of the guard-ship in an atmosphere of petrol fumes and rank tobacco, with a negligible proportion of oxygen and remained well. I have never been seasick since.

I was living in the camp of the Royal Marine Commando in circumstances of the utmost squalor when the surgeon lieutenant on a ship in the Flow, a former student, discovered my presence

68

and invited me to dine. The evening started badly. The captain, who I gather had never asked to meet a civilian guest of the wardroom, invited me to his cabin, whereupon the officers to a man, who had already drink taken, fell flat on their faces. The captain, who was charming, split a bottle of excellent sherry with me and I returned to my hosts in a mood to enjoy the evening. The contrast was overpowering. Instead of walking through ankle-deep mud to a hut furnished with trestle tables and camp chairs to eat a horrible choice of tinned food, I dined at a civilized table with spotless tablecloth and polished silver and food the equal of anything in a London restaurant in time of peace. The wine was especially good.

The trouble came later. We were required to play that deleterious game of Cardinal Puff. By midnight only the Engineer Commander and I were sitting at the table. We carried the others to bed and barely reached ours unassisted.

There was a curious sequel, obviously coincidental. Months later, I was at Marylebone Station making for Aylesbury, when a loud voice shouted from a compartment I was passing. 'Come aboard, Cardinal Puff.' It was the Engineer Commander. I did, and we reminisced about Scapa Flow till I left the train at Aylesbury. That evening I was listening to the radio. In those days the programme was occasionally interrupted by an apparently meaningless phrase that we already knew to be a code message to agents in Europe. Suddenly the radio said: 'Raymond, le docteur Raymond. Ecoutez! Le Cardinal Puff demande encore de biere.' I never knew the explanation, and there probably wasn't one. I knew many agents then in France, but none knew about that game in Scapa Flow, and no one at Scapa Flow knew about my activities with S.O.E.

I began Hitler's war as a blood transfusion officer at Staines, where I was bored and depressed. I hated my separation from my wife and the abandonment of a pleasant private life for an institutional one that I have always loathed. During the 'phoney war' there was nothing to do except to play darts and drink beer at the pub opposite the hospital. We bought a beautiful little

Tudor house at Whitchurch near Aylesbury, where my wife went to live with the bulge that was to become my daughter, and with Agnes my former secretary and Caroline her baby daughter. I tried to transfer from the Emergency Medical Service to one of the uniformed services, but always unsuccessfully. The medical director-general of the Navy was politely interested in what I considered my main qualification, my knowledge of injuries due to cold, but was confident that this would not be a problem for him. He promised to let me know if he proved wrong. Later, when 'immersion foot' became a major problem for shipwrecked mariners, a friend of mine who had never seen a patient with frostbite suddenly blossomed into the uniform of a surgeon lieutenant-commander, and came to London to learn about it from me; he was to be in charge of the whole subject for the whole Navy. The Army was more explicit; I was too old to return to my old regiment as M.O. and not being then a member of the Royal College of Physicians, not highly qualified enough for a specialist appointment. The Royal Air Force was mysterious. The man who interviewed me promised that I would be commissioned in three weeks, but I never heard from him again. In those three weeks I was suddenly transferred to Tindal House, the Middlesex Hospital 'bolt-hole' at Aylesbury, to take charge of the medical wards and teach every kind of medicine to the Middlesex students. I never reminded the R.A.F. of my existence and gratefully settled down to a private life again.

Near Aylesbury lay the manor of Grendon Underwood, a branch of the Special Operations Executive, where young men and girls were intensively trained for intelligence work and sabotage in occupied France. I became part-time medical officer. It was difficult because my patients were always changing their names. It was also an emotional experience. All too often I said goodbye to my patients and knew that I would not see them again. They were dropped by parachute or landed from submarines or fishing boats. Only a few escaped with their lives. One of these was Denis Rake, the bravest man I ever knew.

When I first knew Denis, he kept a little restaurant in Oxford. He did the cooking himself – excellently – and found time to

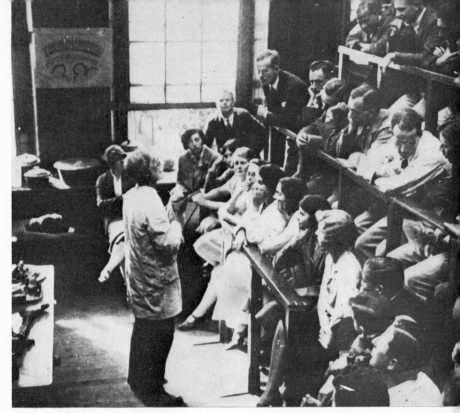

Edinburgh Days
Joseph Ryland Whitaker and his class

Edinburgh Days
Salisbury Crags

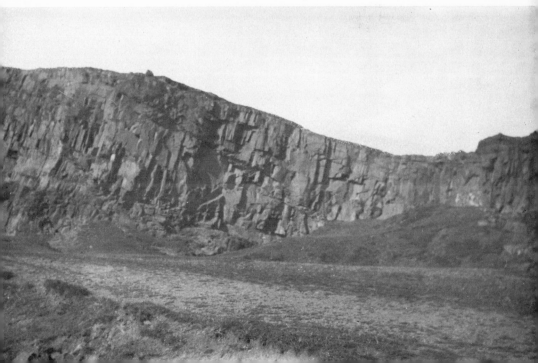

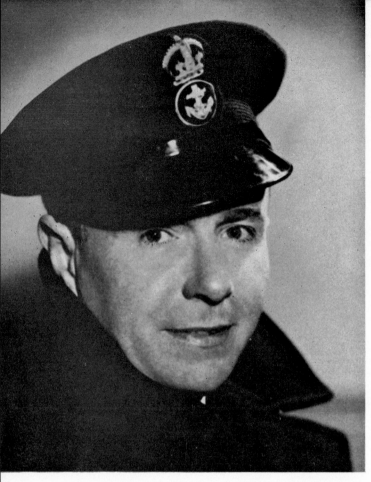

Cloak without Dagger
Denis Rake

Name Dropping
Dr Counsell ('Doggins')

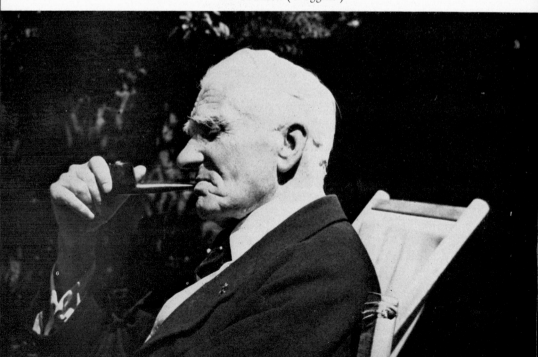

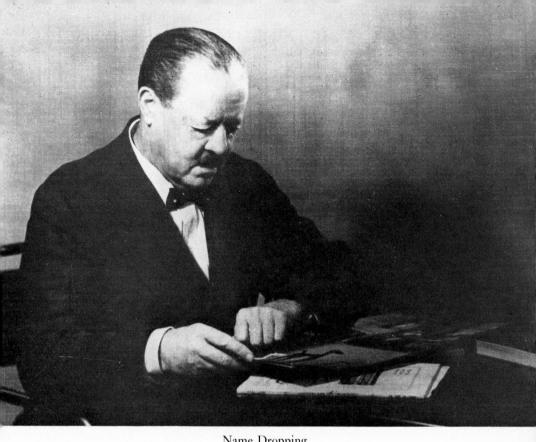

Name Dropping
Brigadier General the Hon. Charles Bruce

Name Dropping
Lliwedd. The scene of many climbs with Frank Smythe

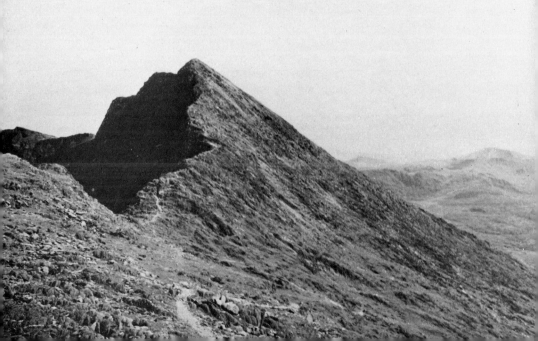

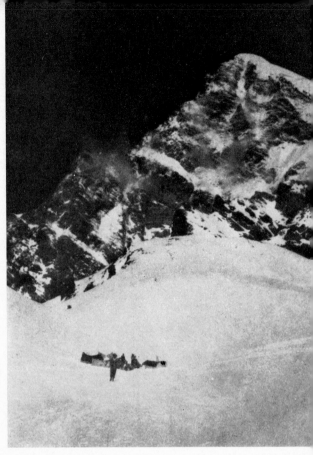

The Kamet Expedition
Kamet

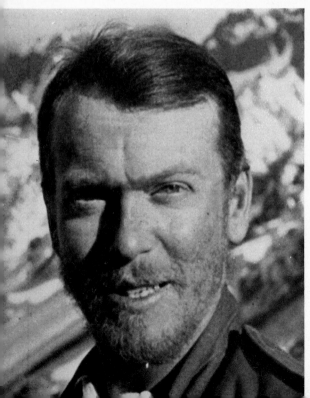

The Kamet Expedition
The author at thirty

talk to his guests too – charmingly. Sometimes he was helped but usually hindered by an ex-monk who suffered severely from acne and religious doubts, and whose name was Desmond. Denis suffered from rheumatism.

He had been born in Belgium of English parents before the Kaiser's war and had suffered much during the German occupation, escaping with difficulty with his mother. His father was executed because of his association with Nurse Cavell. Denis disliked Germans.

In his speech he retained a slightly foreign intonation that drew attention to a manner that was somewhat precious. He affected strange colour schemes and highly scented bath salts. When he felt he knew you well enough he called you 'my dear' a little breathlessly. He was short and plump and no longer young. His walk had a rather feline grace, slightly marred by his rheumatism. He had been a successful singer and dancer under the name of Denis Greer till high kicks became too painful. He cried rather easily.

Although we were almost of an age, I think he promoted me into the post of father. He certainly told me a lot of things about himself which were distinctly confidential. When I left Oxford and moved to London he came to see me sometimes. Then the war came and I heard nothing of him till early in 1940 I got a letter from France – from Sergeant Rake. Then there was silence again until I got a message that Lieutenant Dieudonné had hurt his foot in a parachute jump. And there was Denis.

His French was as good or better than his English and he had become an interpreter in the R.A.S.C. Throughout the 'phoney war' he was stationed at Nantes. In the excitement of the German advance he found himself aboard the *Lancastria*.

His description of the loss of the *Lancastria* was typical. 'My dear,' he said. 'There I was, standing on the deck whence all but I had fled, and I was *entirely* surrounded by *cold water* and you *know* how I've always *hated* cold water; and there was a great big sailor man in the water who kept shouting, "Jump, Den-Den, or you'll get sucked under," and I said, "But, my dear, it looks so *cold*," and he leapt up and clutched at my foot and I fell over backwards and positively *brained* myself, and so I knew no more until I was right out of the cold water and in a boat. Wasn't that *too* lucky?'

He was promptly transferred from the Army into the Navy as an interpreter to the British officers and Free French crew on the mine-sweeper *Pollux*. The ship was mined and once more Denis was dragged from the water. After his rescue he heard a lot of loose talk in a pub about a new organization that was dropping volunteers in occupied France. He strained every effort to find out more about this and in consequence found himself in the War office being interviewed by Colonel Lewis Gielgud, the brother of Sir John. He was transferred back again into the Army, this time with a commission, and before long had embarked on an extensive course of training that led him to Grendon Underwood and back into my care, training in wireless operating, sabotage and parachute jumping.

He was terrified of jumping. Years later he admitted to me that in fact he never had jumped – he was always pushed out. He told me nothing of his work and I asked no questions, until one night in a Buckinghamshire Gethsemane he lay with shoulders shaking with his sobs, and every limb a-twitch with terror, and told me that in a week he was to be dropped alone in France to stay there, always alone, until the end of the war; an end which then seemed very distant to us all. But he would do nothing to back out of it.

Of course, his C.O. knew he was frightened and reported to the War Office. A very important brass hat came down from London next day and asked me what I thought of Donald Duck's condition, for that was his name by then. He was Captain Donald by that time, the name of Dieudonné having been carried long enough for safety. The name D. Rake was just asking for a new pseudonym. I told the Colonel I didn't think his nerves would stand it, but that wasn't what he wanted to know. He had to go – there was no one else to do the job – unless I thought that if he were caught he would blab under torture. I said I didn't know whether I would, so how could I tell whether he would, and added 'and you don't know whether you would'.

Some months afterwards, the War Office discovered that I ought to be paid for my services. I was already a whole-time officer in the Emergency Medical Service and could not accept payment. The whole thing was most irregular and Whitehall was in a flap. After a few months of time and a few hundred-weight of valuable paper had been wasted, I was asked to resign. S.O.E. was furious but Whitehall breathed again. I was now in outer darkness and knew no more of Denis or his colleagues.

But in May 1943, a telegram arrived from Madrid. It read: 'Shall see you soon and need your valuable help. Denis Greer.' I waited, but the weeks became months and I came to believe the worst. Denis had gone back to France, and they had picked him up. I would miss him, for I had come to recognize under his epicene manner something which I didn't remember having met before, a bravery and determination outside my experience.

So for two years I believed him dead, but in September 1945 I had a letter. He was in hospital in Bradford, suffering – believe it or not – from 'rheumatism'.

'I have had a very hard war indeed,' he concluded. 'Once condemned to death and another time to solitary confinement for life, but I'm still here and proudly possess the M.C. I know everyone who knew me is surprised, but I am by far the most surprised.'

Later he arrived in London. He looked older, and there were rather a lot of lines round his mild blue eyes. The dancer's walk was almost obscured by a military strut, but there was a curious new amendment – he limped on both feet. His left chest was ablaze. Beside the M.C., he had the Cross of the Legion of Honour, the Croix de Guerre with Palm, a medal for valour given by the Maquis, and a few campaign ribbons. He was rather shy about it.

In the Rose of Normandy, the story gradually came out, emerged in untidy bits and in the wrong order. He couldn't tell a story for toffee. Even after an hour of hard work, I knew I only had the bare bones of it all.

He hadn't been dropped in France after all. They took him in a warship to Gibraltar and transferred him to a merchantman flying Portuguese colours. He was very shocked by this and refused to sail, so they locked him in his cabin. Somewhere in the Atlantic they transferred him to a submarine which took him to Antibes, and from there to a felucca, from which he had to paddle to shore in a collapsible dinghy.

His adventures henceforward have been told too often to merit repetition. They are told in many books, his own (*Rake's Progress*), Russell Braddon's *Nancy Wake*, E. H. Cookridge's *Inside S.O.E.* and many others. Maurice Buckmaster, the Commander of the French Section of S.O.E. said to me, 'Denis is the bravest man I have ever known.' Nancy Wake said, 'Wherever Denis was, there was laughter.' He was imprisoned and tortured first by the Gestapo and then by the Vichy French, but he got away from both and after a nightmare journey over the Pyrenees with a broken foot, found himself in a Spanish gaol.

The Spanish gaol was worse than the French one. Twelve people of both sexes were crowded into a space large enough for two. They were let out for the purposes of nature only at fixed times. The cell was never cleaned and the food was scanty and bad. As they couldn't all lie down at once, they took it in turns to sleep on the floor, while the rest held bug-killing contests on the walls. Denis had dysentery and thinks he was a little mad. Eventually he was sent to hospital, and it was at this point that I let him down. He got in touch with the British Embassy in Madrid, who refused to do anything for him on the grounds that Denis Rake had been executed by the Germans. Denis was regarded as a dangerous impostor. He thought, perhaps rightly, that a telegram to his own organization would have the same reception, 'but,' he thought, 'if old Greene gets a telegram from me, he will mention it casually to the C.O. No impostor would know of Greene's association with S.O.E. and the C.O. will know that it is really me.' To make matters still more certain, he signed it 'Denis Greer', for no impostor would be likely to know his stage name. He guessed rightly that I would guess the sender of the telegram. He could not know that Whitehall's red tape had ended my association with S.O.E. and that I would never see his colonel again. It never, of course, occurred to me that I was in possession of information which would have been so welcome at that Buckinghamshire manor. I just continued to keep my mouth shut.

One man, Haslam of the British Embassy, had doubts. He and his wife visited him, grilled him and believed him. Haslam came home on leave, visited the S.O.E. H.Q. and made his point. Denis returned to England by air. When the plane touched down at Croydon he fainted. He was soon about again, and the streets of London were the loveliest things he had ever seen. They were battered and grimy but infinitely lovable. But as he walked in them, he developed a curious anxiety to know the time. He would stop strangers and talk to them about it, comparing their watches with his, puzzled if they corresponded, for he was always convinced that his was wrong. It needed months in a mental hospital to get his addled brain to rights again.

At last those taskmasters of his were satisfied. He had done his job. From now onwards there stretched before him a peaceful vista of office work and lectures to the American troops, who had to be taught to hate Germans, often a difficult task. He didn't think he was pulling his weight in the war and volunteered to return. He was landed by Lysander aircraft, and then, in the company of Nancy Wake, there began his most active and dangerous period, culminating in the moment when he, Nancy, John Farmer and the Americans Alsop and Schley, were the first Allied officers to enter the surrendered city of Vichy. It was a far cry from that night with me in Grendon Underwood. Maybe the citation for the cross of Chevalier of the Legion of Honour sums up Denis best. RAKE, Denis Joseph – Captain in the British Army – born in Brussels 22nd May 1901. An officer of the British Army inspired by the highest qualities of courage and perseverance. Parachuted into France (*sic*) for the first time in April 1941, he managed by his skill and daring to establish one of the very first contacts with London. Arrested after being dropped a second time in July 1942, he heroically withstood the most rigorous ordeals of imprisonment and interrogation. Having succeeded in escaping, he was arrested a second time in Limoges. Overcoming the vigilance of his captors, he returned to London after a painful internment in Spain. Parachuted (*sic*) a third time at his own request into the Massif Central district, he took part in all his team's operations. Exemplary in his bravery and selflessness, he gave in every situation the finest demonstration of his devotion to the struggle against the invader. This citation carries with it the award of the Croix with Palm.

But Denis says that's all my eye and Betty Martin.

Like most of the honours that have come to me, the Cross of the Legion of Honour was undeserved and unexpected. Of those I have deserved but not received others must judge; I am not really interested. Perhaps honours are like money; they are not worth while if you have worked for them. The money I have enjoyed has always been 'bukshee'.

I can't remember how or when I became friends with André Lichwitz. Perhaps it was something to do with my short inglorious connection with S.O.E., for André was in England in close association with General de Gaulle. He had been a fashionable physician in Paris and de Gaulle was one of his patients. When the war came he gave up his practice, became a cavalry officer and promised that for the duration he would have only one patient, the General. He proved himself a most gallant officer in the early disastrous years of Hitler's war but eventually retreated, *pour mieux sauter*, with his only patient.

The war over, André returned to Paris and his practice. He was one of the most entertaining of boulevardiers but a serious medical researcher, especially on bone diseases, on which I heard him lecture brilliantly in his hospital. His mistress, who always came to England with him, was one of the most beautiful girls I have ever seen. She was like the young Hedy Lamarr but had prettier ankles. He continued to be the General's doctor and when the state visit of 1960 was planned, André entrusted his great patient's care to me. I was not entirely surprised when my secretary said when I returned from hospital, 'you must ring the French Embassy at once and tell them when you can go.'

Another André interviewed me. Would I take over sole medical responsibility during the state visit? I must not only be in charge of the General's health but make all arrangements for the possibility of an attempt at his assassination. I decided at once that I needed a partner whose French was perfect, which mine was not, and who was a surgeon, and I co-opted my old friend Geoffrey Parker, who had spent much of the war in France, organizing the surgical services of the Resistance and had come back, unharmed after terrifying adventures, as a colonel with a D.S.O. and the Cross of the Legion of Honour.

Arrangements in the event of possible attempts at assassination of the General were obviously the most important. The R.A.M.C. had been advised and, almost at once, the then head of that organization peremptorily requested an interview. I thought that Geoffrey, an ex-colonel, would be better at the job than myself, an ex-lieutenant. He was most co-operative. 'You and Greene need have no worries. The R.A.M.C. will take full responsibility. Leave it all to me.' Geoffrey was not impressed. He replied that I had been put in charge by the French Government and he must consult me before he could be sure that I was willing to hand over my responsibilities. We decided against it.

The Foreign Office telephoned. I replied that having been given these responsibilities I was not willing to hand them over. The F.O. man laughed loudly. 'I thought,' he said, 'that that would be your reaction.' I heard no more from the R.A.M.C.

The first thing was to get from Scotland Yard a complete itinerary of the General's movements. With the extremely efficient help of the ambulance service of the L.C.C. and of Superintendent Gale of the Yard, we arranged for the stationing of ambulances in side streets along all his routes, each to be equipped with blood transfusion apparatus. This was not too easy as the General's blood group was the rather rare A Rhesus Negative. There was a 'let out' here as my own group is O Rhesus Negative which can, if necessary, substitute. Cross-matching would obviously be impracticable. I was therefore continuously in the background. With each ambulance was a police escort and we so ordered things that within twelve minutes of an attack the General could be in the London Clinic, where a suite with operating theatre would be continuously at the ready, with Geoffrey's registrar at the French Hospital in continuous attendance day and night, with nurses from the French Hospital with him. I arranged that specialists in all branches should be continuously on the telephone during the four days of his visit. Lord Evans, Dr Laurent, Mr Langley, Mr Law, Mr Oliver, Mr Battle and Sir Clement Price-Thomas agreed to be continuously in the background.

It was a memorable visit. I was in continuous attendance and despite the General's reputation for aloofness we established an atmosphere of surprising sympathy. Eleanor and I attended the Gala Performance at Covent Garden, when the whole theatre was decorated with tens of thousands of carnations. Under the direction of Dame Ninette de Valois we saw the first act of *Coppelia*, the Market Scene in *Mam'zelle Angot*, Beriosova in *Swan Lake* and Ravel's *Valse*. We lunched with him at the Guildhall, a somewhat embarrassing occasion on which we had to walk the gauntlet between clapping counsellers to the dais. We attended him at a reception, very crowded, very hot, at the French Embassy.

In the four days in which I was almost continuously in his shadow, the General appeared friendly and relaxed. I did not once hear him say 'Non'.

As he boarded the plane to return to France, we were congratulated on our arrangements for his security. We gracefully acknowledged the compliment, but Geoffrey remarked, *sotto voce*, 'But when you remember all we did, it is perhaps a pity that he wasn't just a tiny little bit shot.'

We were concerned again with the General when he paid a private visit to Mr Macmillan at Birchgrove in the autumn of 1961. Geoffrey Parker, Superintendent Gale and I spent a pleasant weekend at the Felbridge Hotel. We did not this time meet the General, who had, we were told, become so bored with security arrangements that he had become somewhat unapproachable. We were however smuggled into Birchgrove.

78

From the window of his A.D.C.'s room I looked up a long grassy slope towards a placid wooded hillside in which there was a conspicuous gap. 'There,' I said, 'is where I would be with my telescopic sights if I meant mischief to the President.' 'You wouldn't,' said his A.D.C. 'There are three Alsatians there.'

Though I didn't meet the General that time he relented to the extent of sending me a very beautiful cigarette case. It's a pity that I don't smoke cigarettes. My poor friend André, a chain-smoker, died that way.

8 Name Dropping

Dr Counsell, 'Doggins' to many generations of Oxford under-graduates had been born in Chepstow in 1863, the son of a civil servant in the Inland Revenue Department. He read medicine at Guy's, married a nurse at twenty-three, and, with the conjoint qualification, went into general practice at Liss. General practice in those days meant more surgery than medicine and one of the best stories of this master raconteur was that of his first (and successful) mastoid, done on a child on the kitchen table by the light of his gig lamp, with tools found in the kitchen drawer. In the midst of a busy practice he somehow found time to take the F.R.C.S. There followed his move to Oxford, where he hoped to specialize as a surgeon; but he arrived at an unlucky time, with no vacancies on the Radcliffe staff for years to come. At first he ran a private surgical nursing home, but the lack of a hospital appointment was bound to tell, and he drifted away from surgery into general practice again. A generation grew up which knew him as a greatly loved physician and observed with a shock of surprise his masterly 'come-back' to surgery in the First World War.

Counsell was a part of all that he had met. To be in Oxford but not of it, was to him impossible. While carrying on a rapidly growing practice, he became an undergraduate of New College, sat every examination without exemption and, disdaining a return to a subject he had already studied, read the honour school of modern history and scored a second. Thenceforward, he threw himself into every university activity, but especially the O.U.D.S. He was largely responsible for its revival after the Kaiser's war and from then until his second eye failed him he was more than the official prompter; he was the friend and confidant of every member and of every visiting actor and actress. His annual party 'after the show' was for many the most important social event of the summer term. There until the dawn actors old and young, with a sprinkling of artists, poets, dramatists, novelists, politicians and even an occasional doctor, filling every chair and sofa, sitting on tables and the tops of bookcases or squatting on the floor, would ply the now almost forgotten art of talk.

The famous O.U.D.S. parties were not isolated occasions. The door of 37 The Broad was always open and no one used the bell. One walked in and shouted 'Doggins' and waited for the genial shout of welcome from the big room with the wide windows which looked across The Broad to the Old Clarendon Building and the decaying stone emperors before the Sheldonian. He must have gone to that house soon after the old emperors had watched the coming and going there of Zuleika Dobson and the Duke of Dorset, and for many years they were able still to see a succession of famous men and lovely women arriving from the ends of the earth or only from the Banbury Road, and to hear them all enter the house in the same informal way. It was only after his sight was gone that the University pulled down the row of beautiful twisted houses which lay between Blackwell's and Holywell, and cast him out to find his way by touch about a newer and less gracious home.

Counsell liked the human race and about its individuals he formed his own opinions, which, whatever others might say, were usually favourable. His tolerance attracted the censure of the more strait-laced, who were shocked to see that, though his own virtue was exemplary, he preferred the company of publicans and sinners. He was intolerant only of the smug and of the Ministry of Health officials. The first he avoided; the second he insulted with subtlety and wit, countering with great skill and infinite enjoyment their attempts to reduce the cost of his panel practice. Nothing was too good for his poorer patients.

He had at one time an enormous practice, but he never had a large income and he died a poor man. Until he took me as a partner in his later years his finances were always in confusion.

He often forgot to send out his accounts and would never send them to patients he greatly liked. 'Oh, my dear chap,' he would say, 'we can't charge him anything. He's such a nice fellow.' When he lent money, which was often, he seldom got it back again because he would always forget about it within a few minutes. He was the despair of his accountant.

In person he was short and slim but well proportioned. His face was ruddy and deeply seamed, even in middle age, by laughter rather than by care. His hair was thick and white and worn rather long for those days. He affected strange garbs, cloaks and big hats and buckled shoes. Such things became him well. They became part of the Oxford landscape. He was the most famous Oxford 'character' of his day, but it is not for his eccentricities that he will be remembered, but for his generosity and tolerance and unfailing kindness.

Charlie Bruce, Brigadier-General the Honourable Charles Bruce, was tough. A boxer, a wrestler, a man of Herculean strength, he had, in his youth, the reputation of a bully. By the time I knew him he was a charming, lovable and intelligent old man, President of the Alpine Club, honorary colonel of the Ghurka Brigade, full of good stories, most of them 'blue'.

He had started soldiering as a subaltern in my own regiment, the Oxfordshire and Buckinghamshire Light Infantry. One night in the mess I was told that in his youth he had bet a large sum that he would run from London to Brighton in a day, stopping for a drink at every pub he passed – there were then no licensed hours – and won. Afterwards I asked him whether it was true. Bruce had a characteristic laugh consisting of a series of violent hisses through the nose. He hissed uncontrollably for some minutes before he was able to say 'Yes', hiss, hiss, 'quite true. But they didn't tell you that I also screwed the barmaid of the Crawley Arms behind the bar. hiss, hiss, hiss.'

One day, long after he was dead, I fell in on Coniston Old Man with a retired colonel who told me a story that I found easy to believe. In the Waziristan campaign his troops were held up by a single pill-box through the slits of which the enemy directed a withering fire. The Brigadier arrived in fury from the rear. He lay on his stomach and moving like a snake across the intervening space, the bullets falling all around him, he broke into the pill-box from the rear. It was too small for the Wazirs to turn their rifles on to him. Five heads were thrown out before the Brigadier, blood dripping from his kukri, strolled back to his troops. I have his kukri.

He was not popular with his superior officers and this was easy to understand. One night when the divisional general was dining in the mess, Bruce became bored and left inconspicuously. Not long afterwards a subaltern rushed in crying, 'Come on you chaps, we're having a great time jumping on the general's tummy.' This was one of his favourite sports. He would lie on his back while a succession of subalterns would take a running jump on to his abdomen. At the moment of impact the great muscles would suddenly contract and the subaltern would be propelled a yard into the air. In his old age he would visit his beloved Ghurkas every year, but he would spend his evenings in the sergeant's mess singing songs and telling dirty stories in the Nepali language.

So the powers that be decided to be rid of him and he was declared medically unfit for further service and warned that he must never walk up a hill again. This was in 1919 and in 1922 he was leader of the second Everest expedition. But his insistence on living his life full out and his phenomenal consumption of alcohol probably did something to bring him to the deplorable medical condition in which he was when, after years of friendship, he decided to put himself in my hands. The decision made, action typically followed. He hailed a taxi in St Mary Abbot's Terrace and drove to Oxford. On my instructions and without argument he gave up alcohol, reduced his weight, took the graduated exercises I enjoined. When, rarely, he took a drink, he would visit me afterwards to confess.

But it was too late. One afternoon at a meeting of the Everest Committee, he referred to the expedition of 1824. Nobody else noticed, or, if anyone did, he did not realize its significance. Knowing that he was the most accurate of men, I glanced at his face. It looked strangely vacant of expression. A few days later his Welsh housekeeper Maggie sent for me. Charlie Bruce had had a stroke of the cruellest kind. He had lost the power of speech and although he was not paralysed, his muscles refused to obey his commands. On one occasion, wishing to clean his teeth, he put the toothbrush in his mouth, struck a match and lit the end of it, all this with no intellectual impairment. Always a man of violent temper, he would smash his crockery and furniture. Only Maggie and I could understand his wishes.

It was four months before his merciful end. He sank slowly towards coma. One day I found him lying peaceably in his bed. He smiled at me but made no attempt at speech. Some inspiration made me say to him in his loved Nepali language, using his nickname amongst his men, 'Sukhi, Bhalu Sahib?' He, who had said nothing intelligible for months, produced his old mischievous grin and very clearly said, 'thik sukhi, mero mitra burho' ('very happy, my old friend'). Soon afterwards the coma deepened and he died.

In my pursuit of Crowley, long before I met him, I followed every clue. In his book, *The Diary of a Drug Fiend* the name of Gwen Otter occurred. I found her in the London Telephone Directory and rang her up. When she answered, I said, 'Do what thou wilt shall be the whole of the law.' She replied, 'Love is the law, love under will. Who the hell's that?' I explained that I was interested in anyone who knew the Beast and she asked me to lunch.

She must have been quite young then, probably about forty, but she looked older. She looked like a little wizened monkey. She was very rich and lived in a charming house, decorated by Marcel Boulestin, in a pleasant Chelsea square. She kept the last of the London salons.

To her everything and everybody was of enormous interest, especially if it or he were scandalous. She was quite uninhibited by convention and many men must have regretted that she was so unlovely. Years later when she was very old and very deaf I took her out to dinner. By this time she talked in a continuous shout that drowned the loud conversation of our fellow-diners.

Looking across at a young couple she remarked, as she thought *sotto voce*, 'Look my dear, at that nice young couple. Why doesn't the waiter hurry with their bill? They are just aching to get to bed.' Later she electrified the company by suddenly shouting, 'I don't see anything wrong with incest. I think it's nice.'

One never called on her in the evening without meeting a celebrity. I remember especially Ernest Thesiger, doing his petit point by the fire, who became a lifelong friend, Turner Layton and Paul Robeson. Long afterwards, knowing that Paul was to sing in Oxford, I invited him to stay in my house. I had no reply. I went to the concert and had just returned when he telephoned from the Randolph Hotel to ask if he could come round. He had not received my letter. He said he was so excited by the applause after his concert that he knew he couldn't sleep. He lay in my long Minty chair and talked entrancingly of his life, of the Negro problem, of all the American problems. Then gradually he came to Negro music and began to illustrate what he said by singing quietly. His voice just filled the room but only just. Then he stopped talking, and just sang. Neither Paul nor I noticed the passing of the hours till suddenly he realized that the sunlight was shining through the curtains and he apologized and left. I never saw him again, but for all his communist activities, I shall remember that night with joy.

Gwen Otter lived to a great age but her end was sad. When her income became too small she lived on capital. She became stone-deaf but never learned to use a deaf-aid. Almost all her friends were dead or had deserted her. She became a bore, telling the same stories of the gay days. Her death was merciful, for she hadn't a shilling left.

Kate Meyrick, the widow of a doctor, was left with a bevy of daughters. I have a vague memory of a son. She became known as 'the night-club queen of London'. Her first and most famous club was Number 43 Gerrard Street in what is now China Town.

'The 43', as it was called, was a remarkable club. It was frequented entirely by the better-behaved young men of the aristocracy and the professional world. There was nothing unruly, ill-mannered or, as we would now say, 'permissive' about it. One could always find there a professional partner of beauty and charm. It might, or might not, be possible to make an assignation elsewhere in the future, but nothing more advanced was permitted there than a discreet kiss or a close embrace on the dance floor. Kate Meyrick saw to that.

I think that 'sex' was more fun in those days. For its full enjoyment there must always be an element of discretion, secrecy and even perhaps a slight sense of guilt and guile. In these days when sexual intercourse has become a public entertainment, much of its pleasure has gone. There were no secret rooms to which one could retire with one's partner. One could not even take her away without Kate's permission, rarely given. She was a mother, albeit a slightly lax one, to her girls. Elegance and discretion reigned.

But otherwise, the laws of the land were regarded as of no consequence. Liquor was sold openly 'out of hours'. The club was regularly raided by the police, usually led by a certain Sergeant Goddard, who, during raids, would imbibe champagne with Kate in her private room. Alas, he ended in prison, but meanwhile had put aside a small fortune from bribes. There was a night when, during a raid, I had the honour of helping the Lord Chancellor of the time to escape through the lavatory window.

My favourite partner was a charming girl whose sights were set very high. A noble lord had asked her for her hand in marriage and she was utterly faithful to him. When he decided instead to marry one of Kate's eligible daughters, all of whom became peeresses, she was genuinely heart-broken. I had the pleasant task of consoling her for a while but she ultimately married a charming but feckless friend. It didn't last. What happened to her I never knew.

The last time I went to 'The 43' was at the end of the General Strike of 1926. I was a special constable and with a colleague presented myself at 2 a.m. at Gerald Road police station to get my orders, only to be told that the strike was over and that we could go back to bed. We had gone to bed early and had no wish to return. We decided, still equipped with armbands and truncheons, to raid 'The 43'. The doorman pushed aside the covering of the little grille and saw my armband. Rapidly the grille was obscured and from within came much sound of clinking glasses and bottles as the evidence of guilt was hidden. Then we were admitted. Kate, looking motherly and respectable received us. 'Raymond, you so and so,' she cried (she never used foul words), and we spent the rest of the night drinking her champagne.

Several books have been written about the remarkable Rosa Lewis. None establishes beyond argument whether she was or was not one of good King Ted's many mistresses. She was undoubtedly available and his appetite for beautiful women – or even women of character who need not have been exceptionally lovely – was insatiable. Who could blame him? One cannot have too much of a good thing.

Her hotel, The Cavendish, was unique. A lot of its spirit was captured by Evelyn Waugh in his early book *Vile Bodies*. What a pity it is that Evelyn did not keep the carefree attitudes of his youth. His early books were the most superbly funny of any written in those wonderful twenties, when we all thought that we had won the war to end war and our one thought was 'on with the dance. Let joy be unrefined.'

At Oxford we didn't like each other much. I was for him too traditional, insufficiently revolutionary. Speaking at the Union we made snide remarks about each other, his being far more clever than mine. Not long afterwards. when I was a general practitioner in Oxford and he a newly successful novelist, we met again and suddenly liked each other. Perhaps we had both changed, Evelyn becoming more serious and I less. We were both frustrated; he could not find time or peace to finish his book *Labels* for which his publishers were pressing him; I was working flat-out in my practice and trying at the same time to prepare myself for a higher qualification. We left the party together, determined to cut our common Gordian knot. We went to stay at the Spread Eagle at Thame, the pub made famous by John Fothergill.

This strange painter manqué, who had been a pupil of Augustus John, had found his true career as an hotelier, had taken over a derelict pub and had made it into one of the most famous hotels in England. It was not only comfortable, with exquisite food, but also had a unique character, with John Fothergill pervading it all. He was an autocrat, as one can see in his book *The Diary of an Innkeeper*. His attitude appealed to many and the undergraduates of his time accepted his dominance and learned much from him about food and wine. Some of us, however, were unwilling to be bullied. One night a lamb cutlet was brought to me on a cold plate and I told the waitress to take it away. Fothergill himself brought it back. 'You ought to know,' he said, replacing it before me, 'that lamb should be served on a cold plate.' I looked him in the eye and said, 'Dear John, you know you are talking balls, but you mustn't talk balls to me. If you don't remove this plate and replace it according to my wishes I shall submit myself to the great pain of breaking it over your head, here, publicly.' He bowed politely and the plate was replaced. At the end of the meal he returned with three very large brandies. 'May I,' he said, 'have the pleasure of drinking a brandy with you, on the house, of course.' We remained friends.

Staying at the Spread Eagle, Evelyn Waugh and I evolved a schedule. We rose at 8 a.m., bathed, dressed, had breakfast and retired to the great parlour, which had a desk at each end. There we worked till lunch-time, at which we ate and drank frugally. Then we went for a long walk over the lovely Oxford countryside, returning in time for a bath and a drink and a good dinner. Then, joining the local yokels in the bar, we drank rather heavily till sleep began to claim us. Day by day we followed this excellent routine.

A copy of Evelyn's first novel *Decline and Fall* – his best, I think – was chained in the first floor loo. One morning Evelyn was late for work. When he arrived in the parlour, I turned and said, 'Can I do anything for you professionally?' 'No,' he said, 'I had just forgotten how bloody funny I could be in those days.'

'Those days'; he was so funny, so easy to talk to, so delightful a companion. A few years later he learned that I was going to

Everest and wrote to me to ask if he could come too, not as a climber but to write a book about our expedition. I was all for it; it would have been a hilarious book. But our own leader had decided, rightly I am sure, that no one should go who was not an experienced mountaineer. I had to turn Evelyn down. I don't know whether he minded greatly and couldn't forgive me, but I did not see him again for many years. The reason for this was more probably his success, which spoiled him. He became a very pompous person and the nearest he could achieve to being a country gentleman. Meeting him at a Heinemann party many years later, I greeted him cordially. He looked up into my face (he was a small man) nodded in an absent-minded way and turned away. I wasn't, I think, important enough for him. I was sorry, for I liked the little man and admired his work.

But I was writing about Rosa Lewis. She has appeared in so many books, including two full-size biographies, that all I need to do is to remind the reader that she started as a beautiful scullion, became the best cook in London, in constant demand at fashionable parties, became the protected darling of many very important men and eventually owned the Cavendish Hotel in Jermyn Street.

The Cavendish occupied the site of the brash and characterless hotel now at the corner of Jermyn Street and Duke Street. It was a long low Georgian building of great charm, full of old sporting prints, rather dimly lit. The food was excellent and the beds (all double) were soft. If a young man booked a room for himself and later turned up accompanied, no questions were asked provided his behaviour was 'comme il faut'. One of the snags of which one needed to be careful was Rosa's hospitality. One was often wafted on one's arrival into her private room, in which a party was always going on, with champagne flowing. The snag was who would pay – never Rosa. As like as not one would find six or more bottles of champagne on one's bill next morning. Once when I stayed at The Cavendish, I was badly overdrawn and rather short of cash. I found all the champagne of the previous evening debited to me; I refused to pay. Rosa was called. 'Rosa,' I said, 'I may wear a good suit but I have no money to entertain your guests, none of whom I had ever seen before.' 'That's all right, dear,' she said, and turning to the cashier, 'put it on Lord R's bill. 'E was too drunk to notice.'

Once, at about ten o'clock in the morning, I was walking down one of the long narrow passages lined with sporting prints when I saw Rosa approaching. She was swaying slightly, and with difficulty holding a glass of rum in one hand and a packet of monkey nuts in the other. The trouble was how to pick out a monkey nut without spilling rum. This problem so completely occupied her attention that she didn't notice my approach. Just before the collision I deftly seized both the rum and the monkey nuts. She was so grateful that she clasped me to her by that time ample bosom. 'What *are* you doing here, dear?' she asked. 'Well, Rosa,' I said, 'I've been spending the night here.' 'I can't think why,' she said. 'It's a bloody awful hotel.'

She led me through a series of rooms along Jermyn Street I had not seen before. We came to a large ornately furnished drawing-room. On a sofa table were dozens of photographs in silver frames, all inscribed to 'My beloved Rosa', often of very well-known faces. She picked up one I didn't recognize and held it for several minutes before her face. 'Lord R,' she said. 'You met 'im last night, you know, the rather tipsy one.' 'Yes, I remember him. He's paying for the champagne. Jolly nice of him, even if he doesn't notice.'

'I stole 'is wallet.'

'Rosa, you didn't! Why?'

'I knew that if I didn't 'e'd go off and look for an 'ore. I didn't want 'im to. You see, if things 'ad gorn right I might 'ave been 'is mother. I'll give it 'im back.'

She kissed the photograph and put it down and we went and had some more champagne, presumably at Lord R's expense.

Hill Wells and I left Oxford together and became students at the Westminster Hospital. We took a lower maisonette in St George's Square and, I can't remember by what means, employed the services of one Bernard as housekeeper, cook, valet, *un homme à tout faire*. He was superb. Small and plump, he had not perhaps the personality of the great Jeeves; he would not, for instance, presume to advise us as to what tie would best go with what suit; but otherwise he was the perfect gentleman's gentleman. The first evening of his arrival my pipe became blocked. I rang the bell and asked whether perchance he had a piece of wire. He, a non-smoker, immediately brought a pipe-cleaner ('Gentlemen, sir, often want pipe-cleaners') and every evening thereafter a pipe-cleaner was laid beside my armchair.

At first we did the shopping ourselves, but Bernard did all the cooking, the conventional English breakfast, tea with home-made cakes, a three-course dinner. We were always out for lunch. He kept the rooms immaculate, cleaned and pressed our clothes and even did our laundry. After a while we turned the shopping over to him and opened accounts at the shops he favoured. At the beginning of each month he would bring us the books and we would give him the cash to settle them.

So passed a glorious year. One evening we returned from hospital to find tea laid as usual. Simultaneously we saw that the cakes were not home-made, but we did not comment, each of us feeling that an adequate explanation would soon be made. Bernard usually made one operation of clearing the tea table and laying the dinner table. The time for the operation came and went. Hill and I looked at each other with a wild surmise and walked down to the basement. There was no Bernard and there were none of his belongings. The kitchen was newly cleaned, the bedroom was empty; everything was in apple-pie order, but there was no Bernard.

The first discovery after this was that our gold evening cuff-links were missing. There was nothing else of value for him to take. Then the demands for payment began to come in; payment for goods for which Bernard had had the cash. A fresh one from the Army and Navy Stores intrigued us for it was from the toy department.

Then a letter from Bernard arrived, full of contrition. He had been in the hands of a widow with children. He had broken loose. Would we take him back? He would repay all.

By this time the police were on his tracks. We told them about the letter but something, some strange public-school inhibition, prevented us from giving them the poste restante address from which he wrote. However, they got him.

Months had passed, months made more devastating by comparison with the heaven that had preceded them. Valets had come and gone, each more incompetent than the last. None was bearable for more than a few days. We sat beside the fire and looked at one another. Words were unnecessary. We just nodded at each other. We must have Bernard back.

Therefore we must save him from prison. We put on our best suits and our most professional manner. We stood up in court, exaggerated our professional status, gave it pompously as our opinion that Bernard was mentally backward, promised to look after him. He was put on probation on condition that he stayed with us for a year. Heaven once more engulfed us.

He was a little resentful at being described publicly as mentally backward, but ultimately realized that St George's Square was more comfortable than Wormwood Scrubs, and anyway, he had no choice in the matter. So passed another peaceful year.

His probation ended and he stood beside our desk. 'Sirs,' he said. 'I am truly grateful to you for all that you have done, but I wish to give notice.'

'But, Bernard, haven't you been happy? What have we done wrong?'

'Sirs, you have been kindness itself. However, I have been studying and have passed my entrance examination to a theological college – I propose to enter the Church.'

I suppose he did. We heard no more of him. Of course I have altered his name. He may be an Archbishop now. I hope so.

Jack Linnell was my predecessor at New End Hospital in Hampstead, both as consulting general physician to the hospital and physician to what was then the London County Council Goitre Clinic. When he went he nominated me, till then his clinical assistant, to succeed him in both posts. There was no nonsense then about advertisement of vacancies or appointment committees. Jack told Sir Alan Daly of the L.C.C. that I was the man for the job and that was that.

He continued to attend the thyroid clinic every Tuesday morning and afterwards we would lunch together at the William IV public house in Hampstead High Street. He often forgot to pay his share. He was always abominably dressed. He died at eighty-nine and left a quarter of a million pounds.

For twenty years we lunched together but he became irritated by the kindly tendency of the inhabitants of Hampstead, so many of whom knew and loved him, to help him across the roads. In the last two years he became weak in the legs, never in the head.

Personally he was not beautiful. He looked like a smaller and fatter Khrushchev, made still uglier by a paralysis of the left side of his face from which he never recovered. In moments of emotion he would weep from his left eye and would not bother to mop his tears. His dentures never fitted and in moments of excitement he would shoot them out beyond his lips, producing a terrifying effect. The chief contradiction lay in the unvaryingly benign look in his bright blue eyes: he never wore spectacles.

His character was complex. In his youth he was a great all-round athlete who just missed several Cambridge blues, but at the same time he was an aesthete with a great knowledge of painting and a happy facility to produce light and epigrammatic verse. He was a man of peace who loved soldiering and had served with great distinction in the Kaiser's war. One who served with him said he should have been given a V.C. several times: he got, in fact, an M.C. and a mention in dispatches. Though he was a very kindly man he never forgot his detestation of the general staff, of whose incompetence and inhumanity he never tired of talking. These contradictions made his conversation fascinating. No one could doubt his intelligence: when over eighty he could read a whole scientific paper as quickly as I could read a page and immediately discuss it with complete understanding. Yet he was utterly illogical: because he had seen the South African troops fighting with great bravery in 1916, nothing that the

South African Government could do half a century later could possibly be wrong.

Till the very end he had a thirst for information about current affairs and he carried on an immense correspondence in a beautiful handwriting that never changed. He remembered among his pen-pals such people as Sir Basil Liddell-Hart, Sir Colin Gubbins, General J. F. C. Fuller and others less famous but equally well informed. In the middle of a discussion he would suddenly stop talking and search through his voluminous and shapeless pockets till he found the latest letter from the man on the spot, which invariably said the last word.

He combined to an apparently impossible degree an intolerance of authority with the most extreme right-wing political thought. In his youth he loved a sortie at night with friends at Scotland Yard and with them was involved in many an enjoyable scrap. Yet his criticisms of police methods and even more of high court judges could be blighting. He liked to remember his occasional contacts with the Secret Service between the wars. That branch of Government could do no wrong.

To the end his mind remained acute and his memory phenomenal. Only his legs reflected a gradual deterioration. With his intellect still undimmed he simply fell asleep and after a fortnight in a coma peacefully departed.

Had it not been for Frank Smythe I would never have seen the Himalaya. I was never a first-class climber on rock or snow, but I was a moderate one on both, and sometimes a reliable second-rater in all circumstances is more desirable as a companion than a man who is a tiger on the one and a rabbit on the other. I had two other advantages: I was a doctor and I was physically very strong.

I cannot now remember when I first knew Frank Smythe. We were two small boys in a small town who met casually at children's parties and were only vaguely aware of each other's presence. We went afterwards to the same school, Berkhamsted, and there I begin to remember him more distinctly, a rather frail fair-headed boy who was said to have a weak heart and was not allowed to play football because of a murmur in the chest which the doctors of those far-off days believed to have some sinister significance. He still had it when I examined him twenty years later in the Himalaya, and he still looked incongruously frail. I did not know him well at school, for we were in different houses, and on different 'sides', and a double gulf lay between us, across which we could do no more than grin at one another rather shyly.

I think that these two facts influenced his whole life; the mistaken diagnosis which set him apart from his fellows and implanted a determination to prove his physical strength; the consequent interference with his early schooling, which planted him for a time under the care of an ignorant and masochistic parson and sent him to Berkhamsted with an intellectual handicap. Physically on his mountains, intellectually in his books, he tried always to reach heights which were just a little beyond his powers, great though these were.

We both began climbing when we were still at school and from that time mountains were what he really lived for. But although we had known each other for so long, it was only in the early twenties that we met by chance on the top of Gimmer Crag, both of us pursuing the 'reprehensible pastime' of solitary climbing, which we both continued, but less than before this chance meeting. After then we met often in Wales and in the Lakes. We amused ourselves in our own way, climbing mountains without looking up the routes in the guide-books and afterwards infuriating the serious climbers by our inability to explain or to name the routes we had taken. One of our favourite quotations was about the great pioneers of rock-climbing J. M. Archer Thomson and A. W. Andrews, the authors of the guide to Lliwedd, the fearsome cliff beside Snowdon.

> *The Climber goeth forth to climb on Lliwedd*
> *And climbeth all the ways that man hath trod,*
> *But which of all the thousand ways he doeth*
> *Is known alone to Thomson and to God.*
> *(And, of course, Andrews!)*

I never climbed with him in the Alps and although we met so often I do not think I ever really got to know him until he invited me to join him in the Himalaya in 1931. We decided to climb the first '25,000-footer' ever to be ascended and we fixed on Kamet, a mountain 25,447 feet high, which lies in a not too inaccessible position at the end of the Zaskar Range, which runs northward from the main Himalayan chain. Kamet had the advantage of being in British territory, though it lies only a mile from the Tibetan frontier. The way there was well worked out, as there had been ten previous attempts. Indeed the great Himalayan explorer C. F. Meade had himself made three attempts and had got within 2,000 feet of the top.

At great altitudes a new force seemed to enter into Frank. His body, still apparently frail as it had been in boyhood, was capable of astonishing feats of sudden strength and prolonged endurance. His mind, too, took on a different colour. At sea-level the mistaken sense of inferiority so unfairly implanted by his early experiences rendered him sometimes irritable, a little tactless and rather easily offended. At high levels, the self-confidence which flowed into his mind and body, the emanation, as it were, of the mountains whose strength he loved, changed him almost beyond recognition. It seemed impossible above 20,000 feet to disturb his composure or his essential quietism. I remember the Kamet Expedition as a period of calm unbroken by more than a rare small ripple of disagreement, and the calm was the result of Frank's confident but always modest and unassuming leadership.

9 The Kamet Expedition

None of us was rich, and expeditions to the Himalaya cost a lot of money. There is first of all the equipment to be bought: special climbing clothes for great heights, tents, ropes, cooking things and tinned food, and all the thousand and one oddments you need when you are entirely out of touch with shops and indeed all human habitations, for weeks on end. Then you have to get yourselves and your equipment all the way to India in ships that are delightful but certainly not cheap. Once in India you have to engage native porters and pack animals to carry all your stuff; and their wages, though very small, mount up astonishingly. There were various ways of paying for all this in 1931. You could collect the seeds of rare plants and sell them in England for very gratifying sums. Smythe reported in *The Times*, the finding of a glade of white peonies on the way to Kamet. Weeks later in camp on the lower slopes we saw, still miles away, a small figure running. We watched him hour by hour toiling up the valley. He carried a yellow envelope addressed simply to 'Smythe, India'. The telegram read 'Bring seed white peony expense no object'. Unfortunately, by seed time we were far away on the other side of the range. Another way of paying was to take a cinema film, which was profitable but irksome and this we did. The best was undoubtedly to get the support of *The Times*, whose readers in those days had apparently an inexhaustible appetite for other people's excitements.

Our ultimate aim was Everest, the highest mountain in the world. Seven years had gone by since Mallory and Irvine had left their camp on its upper crags and, after an instant's view through a cloud-rift, had disappeared for ever. No one then knew whether they had reached the top, but every young climber wanted to know – to give them the honour if they had succeeded or to succeed himself if they had failed. But Everest lies in Tibet. The Tibetans were a people who had isolated themselves from the rest of the world, not because of any silly superstition but from a wise and far-sighted policy. The rulers of Tibet could see a haystack at ten yards as clearly as any of us. They had looked at what we call European civilization and, quite frankly, they didn't like it very much. They had no roads or railways, no telephones, no radio or TV sets, no newspapers and no plumbing or sanitation, but they also had no traffic problems, no propaganda, no stock exchanges, no pop music or professional comedians and, apart from an occasional frontier incident, no wars. They preferred to live in poverty and peace and to isolate themselves from the contagion round them. They did it very thoroughly. They did not let foreigners in without a passport, which sometimes took years of persuasion to get, and very wisely the Government of India respected their hesitation and discouraged anyone from trying to gate-crash the forbidden land. Alas that the Chinese later showed fewer inhibitions. Meanwhile there was Kamet.

The first time we saw Kamet it was a hundred miles away. It was very early in the morning and we were asleep on a verandah at Ranikhet, a little town in the foothills of the Himalaya. Frank Smythe saw it first and woke us. Without getting out of bed we could see a mist beyond the garden. The mist was green with the filtered light of the forests in the valley below. Then came ridge after ridge of rolling pine-covered hills, and at last, apparently hung high in the blue sky above them, the edge of a silver saw. One tooth was bigger than the others – that was Kamet.

We didn't see it again for weeks, because it was always hidden by nearer mountains. Those weeks were filled with delightful wandering through valleys thick with flowers; climbing over high grassy downs and barren ridges; and clambering along the cliffs of deep ravines.

There were nights when our small green tents were pitched in meadows of purple iris, and others when the wind tried to blow them from narrow platforms cut in the hard snow of high mountainsides – until, where the narrow path we had followed turns suddenly northwards and upwards over the edge of India into Tibet, we saw our mountain again. It looked rather forbidding at close quarters, towering nearly 10,000 feet above our heads. On the left a precipice fell very steeply from the summit ridge – an obviously unclimbable place – and on the right the face was covered with a glistening surface of ice up which it would be necessary to cut steps laboriously for days, work too hard at that height where the thinness of the air makes every movement difficult. But between the two there lay steep snow slopes which looked possible. They fell away to a snowy col where a camp could be pitched in a position free from the fear of avalanches. We called it Meade's Col.

The way to the col was guarded by a wall of rock and ice a thousand feet high. It took us several days to find a way up and four camps were pitched between our base and our last camp on the col. As you climb higher, the air grows steadily thinner and your breathing gets faster and more difficult, but you can get used to this by taking time, climbing only about a thousand feet in a day and then pitching camp and waiting till you have got used to the new altitude. At first the smallest movement makes you exhausted and breathless. It's an effort to do up a bootlace or turn over in your sleeping bag. But gradually strength returns and the next day another thousand feet can be climbed almost as easily as the last.

At the camp on the col there was not room for the whole party, so while Smythe, Shipton, Holdsworth and Lewa our sirdar made their successful attempt, we others watched them from the camp below. When our turn came, Beauman, who should have been our leader, was too mountain-sick to start, but Birnie and Kesar Singh, our best porter, and I left the camp at six forty-five, as soon as the sun had thawed our frozen tents, and began the slow trudge towards the summit. At this height, 23,000 feet, you start tired out. Every step was an effort, and between each step we had to pause for two complete breaths, but we didn't stop, for fear of being unable to start again. So for three hours we toiled slowly upwards – step, breathe; breathe again, step, breathe, breathe again – keeping the rhythm going steadily. The work, of course, falls chiefly on the leader who has to make the steps in the snow, and after three hours I was done. Birnie took the lead, but somehow I couldn't adjust my rhythm to his. I felt sick and exhausted. I decided to stay where I was, and sent on the other two without me.

It was a sunny, windless morning. I took off the climbing rope and lay down in the snow and basked happily. White snowfields and red precipices stretched far away until they merged into the brown upland of Tibet. Two hundred and fifty miles away, the Karakoram mountains lay on the horizon. Looking almost as far away, the little green tents of home were clustered at my feet. I felt happy and comfortable, and I went to sleep.

An hour later I woke up feeling very energetic. The top of the mountain looked very near and glistened invitingly in the sunshine. I told myself that it was too late to make the summit and that I would go on just a little way and meet the others on their return journey. In a little tangle of crevasses I lost their tracks, and the shape of the mountain hid them from view, but I kept near the edge of the great eastern precipice and made good progress.

Three hours passed. Now the slope was steeper, and I had no idea where my companions were. Some 300 feet above me was a white ridge in full sunshine. I thought if I could get thus far I would be able to see the top and relieve what was beginning to be a gnawing anxiety for their safety. The way became excessively steep, and the snow dangerous, a shifting powder a few inches deep on hard ice. Once the surface slipped, probably only a few inches but enough to alarm me. Here a serious slip would have meant a fall of some 7,000 feet down the eastern precipice. I felt quite confident about stopping myself, but the others were less experienced and my anxiety grew. I gave a shout and heard a cheerful and unintelligible noise above. Almost at the same moment I saw their tracks. I cut across to them and turned upwards again towards the ridge I had picked as my look-out.

Then suddenly my head rose above the ridge and my eyes,

expecting a further snowfield and yet another ridge, saw for one moment nothing. Then casting them down, I saw a sea of white cloud stretching without interruption to the purple horizon. A few yards to my right lay the summit, and coming from it towards me Birnie and Kesar Singh.

It was four in the afternoon when we began the long descent. I remember that once Kesar Singh slipped and that Birnie seemed to wake for a moment, hold him on the rope, and relapse again into sleep-walking. This is the most dangerous part of a long climb, and during this time I think I kept my wits and my balance. But when the snowfield near the camp was reached I began to fall at almost every step. I noticed that I had stopped falling before I noticed the reason – that Holdsworth had come out from the camp and was half-leading me, half-carrying me, towards my tent. A few minutes later, just twelve hours from the start, I was in my sleeping bag drinking rum out of a tin mug. I enjoyed that rum.

Camp V was no place for a rest cure. The night following the ascent of Kamet by the second party brought to many of us our first experience of a Himalayan wind. Icy blasts of terrifying velocity shook our small tents and, creeping through the flaps, froze the noses of the climbers. But they snuggled deeper into their sleeping bags and slept once more the dreamless sleep of exhausted men.

The very next morning a move was made to lower and warmer places. A somewhat dilapidated party broke camp and moving slowly on frost-bitten feet wound its way through the great ice-fall which separates the sites of Camps IV and V. At Camp IV we stayed long enough to have lunch and pack up our belongings, then continued our downward way. It led down the great mountain face of rock and ice on which, for the sake of laden porters, we had fixed ropes on our upward journey. On our return the porters were not alone in their dependence on them. One of them, designed to round several corners, was of necessity very loose. Disturbed by the movements of the man ahead of me, it chose the moment at which I was most trustful to leave the mountainside and dangle, quivering with apparent glee, in space.

I also dangled. The rope firmly clutched in my right hand, my ice axe in my left, I was dangling from the only part of the route from which a man could dangle. With an effort I succeeded in swinging back on to the mountain and kicked and scrambled wildly into safety. Such effort at such an altitude carries its punishment. For ten minutes I lay and panted before I could continue on my way to the comparative comfort of Camp III at 20,600 feet.

On the following day we descended a couloir to Camp II and early on June 26th in fast falling snow and a bitter wind we began the double march to Base Camp. My frost-bitten toes made walking painful, and I felt old and tired. The wind seemed to find its way through every chink and buttonhole of one's clothing and the snow fell so fast that no sight of distant mountains diverted one's attention from present misery. In the neighbourhood of our old Camp I the snow began to fall less thickly and far ahead we could see the end of the East Kamet Valley and the dark and snow-streaked rock peaks lying above Base Camp. How gladly one would have walked, with what an added spring in one's step if, instead of that comfortless stony place, the end of our journey had been a Lakeland farm or a little English pub, with sandy floor and glass-ringed bar and polished tankards in a row and upstairs the soft bed we felt we deserved.

It was at this point, at about, I suppose 16,500 feet, that a change came over my feelings. Haldane has written how, in his experiments on the effects of low air pressure, he sat in his steel cylinder with the pressure gradually rising towards the normal; and how, at a certain 'level' the electric light glowed suddenly more brightly. At first he thought that the current had been increased, but later he came to realize that the change was in himself and not in the current. For me, not shut in a steel chamber but walking slowly down the East Kamet Glacier, depressed by wind and weather and hobbling on painful feet, the whole aspect of life suddenly changed. I began once more to appreciate the pleasures my senses brought me. My feet were just as painful, but they mattered less. I was just as tired, but my weariness only accentuated the pleasure with which I anticipated

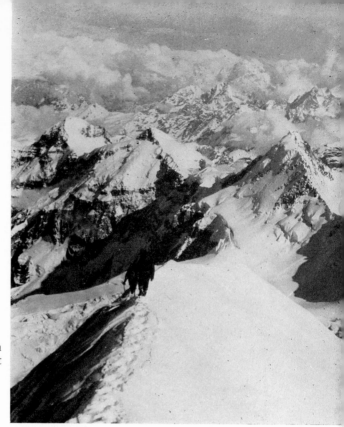

The Kamet Expedition
The summit of Kamet

The Kamet Expedition
Badrinath

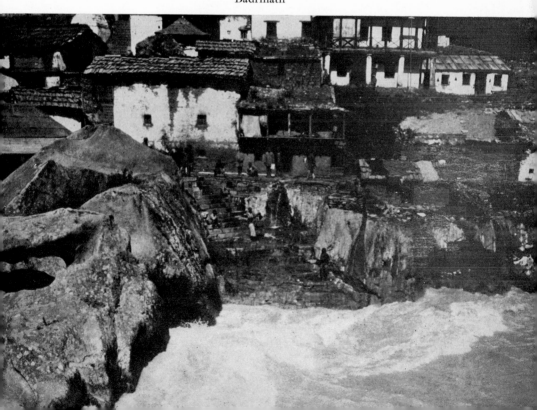

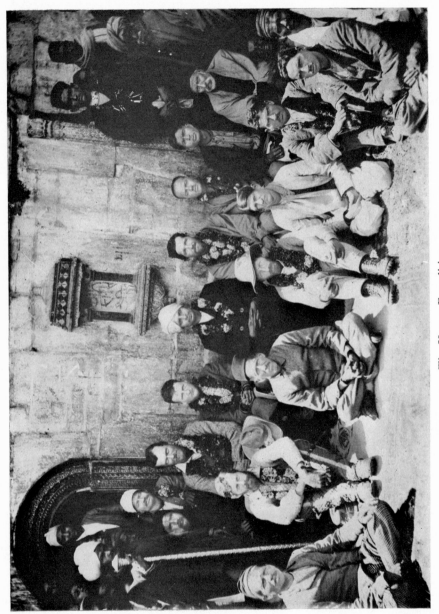

The Kamet Expedition
The members of the expedition with H.H. The Rawal Sahib of Badrinath

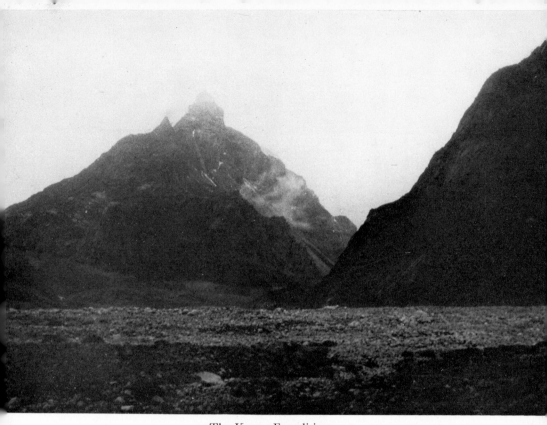

The Kamet Expedition
The source of the Ganges

Journey to Tibet
Mrs Wrangham – Hardy's Elephant

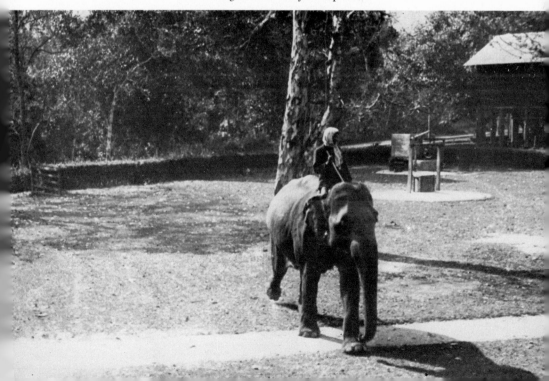

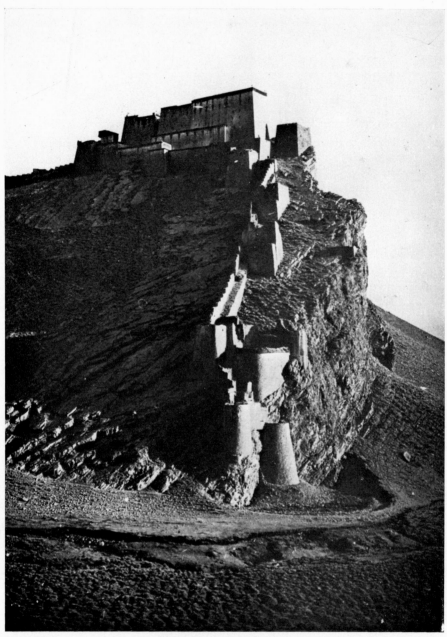
Through Tibet to Everest
Khamba Dzong

the comforts of what I now regarded as the little safe home on the moraine which lay ahead. The peaks beyond the Raikana Glacier seemed to come nearer. The snow over which I dragged my tired feet was whiter and more scintillating, and when, little by little, blue patches began to show between the clouds they seemed a brighter blue than the skies of Kamet. The sinking sun, shining through broken racing clouds, gave a more homely light and the lengthening shadows on the snow seemed like the shadows of the Cumbrian Hills.

It is clear that not only are our senses dulled by lack of oxygen, so that the light in the steel chamber seems dull and the blue of the Himalayan sky less bright, but that all one's mental processes suffer the same fate. Especially at great altitudes one cannot gloat over one's pleasures. One loses, as Goethe put it, 'the courage to submit to impressions; to be delighted, touched and exalted'. But now this courage was suddenly restored, and I continued my way down the glacier savouring with slow care the impressions I received from eye and ear and nose. In the last three weeks the moraine had largely lost its coating of snow on bare boulders. Life had begun. The change was thrilling to eyes which for those three weeks had seen no green but the pale aniline of our tents. Grasses were beginning to sprout between the stones and a saxifrage was almost in flower. A great apple-green moss was spreading over the boulders. The wind up in the valley smelt of distant vegetation and had lost the cold virginity of the winds of the high places. Water flowed again and the hills lost their silence, a strained silence broken only by the occasional crash and moan of an avalanche.

And at last the Base Camp lay in sight below us, smoke rising from its kitchen, no comfortless and stony place, but a cheerful home with a cook to make our meals, and rum and a gramophone, and round it masses of yellow daphne, the scent of which was blown up towards us by a warm breeze as evening fell.

We were not content with the ascent of Kamet. The full story of our wanderings was told by Frank Smythe in *Kamet Conquered*. The monsoon seemed momentarily at rest and the weather was sunny. The deep snows of our ascent had melted and the way was beset with little brooks bubbling over red pebbles and resting a while in quiet pools in which we bathed. Flowers were everywhere. Sometimes the babbling brook changed unaccountably to a fierce torrent across which we had to make our way by scrambling along a tight-rope. The yaks that carried our luggage were less lucky. They were forced into the torrent and swept away, but struggling yakfully reached the farther shore. The yak, despite its ungainly appearance is enormously agile.

Our next objective was the holy city of Badrinath, seat of the Rawal Sahib, the pope of Hinduism. We could have taken a long but easy route down the Dhaoli valley to Joshimath and thence by the well-worn pilgrim route. We decided however to cross the Zaskar Range, over which lay only one pass, the Bhyundar Kanta, 16,700 feet high. Its first recorded crossing was in 1862 and only two crossings had since been made, one by Doctor Tom Longstaff and one by Charles Meade early in the century.

It was on the way there that Frank Smythe began to have toothache. For several days he bore it with only an occasional grumble, but on his birthday, at a place called Eri Udiar, he at last capitulated and asked me to extract the tooth. Unfortunately my chloroform and local anaesthetics had been sent down with our heavy luggage to follow the easy route to Badrinath: I had only my morphine. I gave Frank a shot and left him to carve a dental prop out of juniper root. When I returned I found him unduly cheerful: to give himself Dutch courage he had consumed more than half a bottle of rum. I extracted the tooth and Frank, after one screamed expletive, passed into oblivion. We carried him to his tent at about six in the evening and he slept quietly until I retired to my tent at about nine o'clock. At about two in the morning, I was awakened by a curious noise and, emerging in pyjamas only in a temperature well below zero Fahrenheit I found that Frank's head was protruding from the flap of his tent, his neck supported by one of the ties. He had apparently decided that he was going to be sick, had got his head out just in time, but had not the strength to withdraw it and was strangling. When I rescued him from this predicament he stopped breathing. I gave him artificial respiration but every time I rested for a moment he stopped again. After two hours, spontaneous breathing returned. Luckily the hard exercise involved prevented me from freezing solid. Within a few hours he was well, wide awake and demanding breakfast, but he suffered for a week from 'Saturday Night Paralysis' of his right arm.

I have only twice operated under anaesthesia at great altitudes. The other occasion was two years later on the way to Everest. As two aeroplanes have been known to collide in an otherwise empty sky, so the ponies of Paul the interpreter and Lobsang Tsering the postman collided on the open plain with such violence that both lay momentarily stunned in the dust. Paul was the first to recover and with no injury but a broken little finger galloped into camp. Willy McLean and I cantered back six miles before we found Lobsang, conscious now and nursing a broken collar bone. With the arm in a sling he was capable of riding back. In camp I gave him a mere breath of chloroform while Willy reduced the fracture. Suddenly heart and lungs stopped acting simultaneously. I filled a syringe with Coramine, struck for the heart and began external cardiac massage while Willy applied artificial respiration. Lobsang's heart soon began to beat again and respiration returned. Within an hour he was smoking a cigarette. I don't know which part of our treatment worked but I've had a weakness for Coramine ever since.

Mumm, the great Himalayan explorer, had suggested that there was a pass from the head of the Banke Valley over to Badrinath, but no one had ever explored the valley to its head. Beauman and I set out to do this. On the way we followed a line of apparently human tracks that our porters identified without hesitation as those of a Yeti, an 'abominable snowman'. He was called the badmanch in those parts. The curious thing about these tracks was that after we had followed them for an hour or two they suddenly stopped. We concluded that they were not in fact those of a Yeti but of our guardian angel who had grown tired of leading two mortals who were annoyingly in no need of his protection and had flown away. There was no pass. The head of the valley was hemmed in by a wall of peaks like the aiguilles of Mont Blanc. The face of the valley was a sheer wall of ice plastered with hanging glaciers that persistently discharged great avalanches into the glacier below. Being no heroes we returned discomfited.

The badmanch or Yeti was well known to the porters. There were two varieties, one small and harmless, almost certainly a kind of ape. The other was larger, more human in aspect, walking always on its hind legs. The female had breasts so long and pendulous that when she had to run she would knot the nipples behind her neck. I told this later to my brother Hugh, then recently returned from Malaya where he had served on the staff of General Briggs. 'Oh yes,' he said, 'we had those in Malaya, but there she used to sling her breasts sideways to knock people off bicycles.'

The ascent to the Bhyundar Khanta Pass was unpleasant in the extreme. The sun had disappeared and the rain of the valley below had turned to sleet. There was a thick mist and a biting wind. The visibility was down to a few yards. The way would have been difficult to find in the best conditions. By good fortune we struck the lowest point of the pass and began the descent through wet mist into the Bhyundar Valley.

Suddenly everything was changed. We were below the clouds at last and the valley lay before us carpeted with flowers. The flowers grew in such profusion that the valley floor looked as though covered with brightly coloured handkerchiefs. We waded ankle-deep in primulas, wine-red potentillas, purple irises, forget-me-nots, borage, blue poppies, huge yellow lilies, orchids of all colours, green fritillaries, pansies, geraniums, more flowers than we could name. Every step crushed a dozen. In this garden we camped beside a brook. It was hard to leave the Valley of Flowers.

The Khanta Khal Pass led us through thick jungle, in which sometimes we were forced to go on hands and knees, cutting our way with our kukris, to the Alaknanda valley, the main source of the Ganges, and the pilgrim route to Badrinath.

106

There we were no longer alone. Pilgrims cluttered the path, wealthy ones borne in their palanquins; poor ones walking slowly, their wives sweating behind them carrying their children, their scarce food and their household goods. Some obstructed the way by measuring their length upon the ground, rising slowly, lying down again, as they had done for many weeks since they left the plains. Everywhere dirty imploring hands solicited alms. We crossed a crazy bridge that seemed to consist only of a cat's cradle of string overlaid with rotten wooden planks, through which we could see the plunging Alaknanda, and arrived in Badrinath. There the most important product on sale was one called Shilazit, the panacea for all ills, capable of curing all known diseases and, moreover, of making old men young and young men crazy. Though the Rawal Sahib was the local equivalent of the Pope of Rome, it cannot be said that his palace could vie with the Vatican or the shrine of Vishnu with St Peter's. Perhaps it was as well, for we were dirty, ragged and unkempt. Nevertheless the Rawal Sahib greeted us graciously, hung garlands of flowers about our necks, was photographed with us and gave us handsome presents of mangoes, nuts, onions and goa.

Our plan was to explore the Badrinath Range, rarely visited and never competently mapped. We rested a while in the village of Mana, whence the poor remnants of an old trade route climbs over the Mana Pass into Tibet. The path along the Sarsuti Valley was still in good condition, but the valley is so narrow that huge blocks of stone fall frequently into the raging torrent below. One missed me by inches. I remember the incident because I was thirty at the time and I had had the curious experience of being told by three fortune-tellers that I would die at thirty. One, ten years before, had predicted this from my palm: one more recently had told it from the cards: one had told it from the stars. All were nearly right, but not quite.

Above the gorge, the Sarsuti Valley was dull, featureless and filled with thick mist. We camped on a lawn at the junction of the valley with the Arwa. The mist had cleared and the valley floor was carpeted with flowers. There was a lovely pool into which despite the expostulations of the porters, I plunged. The cold was intense and as my body struck the water I was suddenly reminded of an experiment we had made at school to demonstrate the phenomenon by which one can lower the temperature of still water below the normal freezing point: shake the flask and the water suddenly becomes solid. Happily it didn't, but I lost no time in my return to the bank.

In the Arwa Valley reality corresponded not at all with the maps, the makers of which had wisely decided to trust to guess work rather than risk their lives in producing accurate maps of a region that would be visited by so few that their efforts would be wasted. Indeed no records existed of anyone before ourselves who had been so unwise. But the weather had cleared. The valley was full of stones and we progressed by only six miles on our first day.

We were in perfect physical condition and could climb, at over 17,000 feet, at alpine speed. With Smythe, Shipton and our Sherpa Nima Dorje, I climbed an easy peak of some 19,300 feet and basked on the summit for several hours. Meanwhile Beauman, Birnie and Holdsworth had ascended the southern fork of the valley and found an admirable camping site at 19,000 feet. In the distance the summit of Kamet dominated the view, glowing red in the evening light.

The next day was one of glorious climbing under a hot sun and ended on the watershed of the Alaknanda and Gangotri rivers, never previously seen. The party split at this point, small parties attacking each its own peak. Eleven were climbed, all previously unnamed, all over 19,000 feet. We crossed five passes. On the descent from one we called the Avalanche Peak (21,800 feet), Smythe was carried away by an avalanche but survived with a broken rib. On that day Beauman and I ascended a rock peak of 20,500 feet that stood out boldly from the glacier near the camp.

It was decided that Birnie and Smythe should cross a pass of some 20,000 feet and explore the glaciers on the Gangotri side of the watershed. Shipton and Holdsworth were to continue climbing the neighbouring peaks. Beauman and I were to descend to

Mana and explore the upper reaches of the Alaknanda to the source of the Ganges. In the event Beauman decided to remain at Mana. Smythe, partially incapacitated by his broken rib that made impossible the deep breathing so necessary at great altitudes, decided to come with me to the source of the Ganges.

The floor of the Alaknanda Valley was of soft turf dappled with gentians, but the walls were gigantic and of granite. Here and there were caves in which hermits had lived or perhaps still lived, for in the absence of sanitation we thought it wise to inquire no further. The lawn gave place to a stony waste through which flowed a torrent that we had to cross. Attempts to find a bridge of snow all failed, so Smythe and I were forced to ford it, saved from being swept away by a rope from above. When once a rope had been fixed the passage should have been wet but easy, but one of our porters, known as the egg-wallah for his skill in extracting eggs from unwilling sellers, lost his foothold and was swept from the rope. In horror we saw him swept away down one fall after another as we raced helplessly beside him. It seemed obvious that he was dead by drowning or concussion, but after several hundred yards he was swept into a pool from which I pulled him, naked but unharmed. But the eggs were lost.

We camped in a grassy hollow below Nilkanta, perhaps the most beautiful of all Himalayan peaks. In the evening Smythe and I left the little camp and scrambled diagonally up the hillside above. It was dark below, but Nilkanta stood above us, more precipitous than the Matterhorn seen from Zermatt, bathed in the evening light.

From our camp our way was through a wilderness of boulders through which the Alaknanda wound a tortuous way. Sometimes we were forced to climb the steep cliffs through which it had cut its way, descending again to dells bright with flowers or filled with snow. At last we came to a scene of utter desolation where the river, the main source of the Ganges, burst from beneath a dirty snout, the combined end of the Bhagat Kharak and Satopanth Glaciers. There was no beauty here but an impressiveness about the scene, huge precipices dimly seen through swirling mist, a world of vast tumbling boulders, with no sound except the roar of the torrent that would one day become 'the slender thread of a lotus flower' and finally the most famous river of the eastern world. Here, driven by some strange impulse, four men washed themselves, two Christians and two Bhuddists, to none of whom Vishnu was more than a name.

We descended to Badrinath and on the way rejoined our friends. We were received with much ceremony by the Rawal Sahib, who gave to Smythe and myself the rank of Mahatma in recognition of our wetting (hardly to be described as bathing) in the source of the Ganges. He explained through an interpreter that by our action we had washed away not only all our past sins but also our future ones, a dispensation of which I regret to say I have taken too little advantage. I still treasure the little brick of baked Ganges mud that is my ensign.

On our former visit we had seen little of Badrinath. We now pitched our tents in a flowery pasture well away from the bustle and odours of the holy place. It is not an attractive one and my chief memory of it is of vast areas of corrugated iron, but the temple itself is ancient and picturesque. Throughout the whole of the Orient one is assailed always by this paradox, the beauty of ancient art and the vulgarity of all things new. The Rawal himself showed us his temple, the shrine of the sacred image of Vishnu, a small idol about three feet high of black marble covered in gold drapes. The idol is well fed, a sumptuous meal once a day. Near by is an enclosed bathing pool fed by a hot spring. Though spiritually greatly inferior to a wash in the source of the Ganges, a bathe here is considered to bring much credit. Better still is to descend the smooth wet steps to the river itself and there to immerse the body in the torrent, clinging to an iron stanchion. Sometimes less able worshippers are swept away.

It was our last camp among the high Himalayan peaks. We were rewarded by a sight of Nilkanta by moonlight and the next morning we saw the mountain again, bathed in the morning light. All that now remained was a slow progress down the pilgrim way to the hospitality and civilization of Ranikhet.

10 Journey to Tibet

Everyone now knows that Everest is the highest mountain in the world, first climbed in Coronation Year, 1953. To me one of the most memorable headlines of all time was the *News Chronicle*'s 'All this and Everest too'. On the preceding Friday afternoon someone at the BBC telephoned and explained that he wanted me to appear on television and announce the ascent. 'But it hasn't yet been climbed.' 'No, but it might be over the weekend and then where would we be? You *must* record a talk tonight. Just in case.' 'But I can't.' 'Why?' 'Because it is an invariable rule that as soon as I finish work on Friday I drive my family to my house at Whitchurch – that is my wife, my two children, the *au pair* girl, the budgerigar, the dog, the cat and probably a newt or two. I can't disappoint all these people, especially the newts. You should have thought of this yesterday. I could have done it last night.' A long argument ensued, ended by the question 'Did you say you were going to Whitchurch? How far is that?' 'Forty-five miles.' 'May I send a recording van there tomorrow?'

The van came and was parked in my curtilage. Many little men ran from it with large cables, over the terrace, through the window, into the library. There a large apparatus was installed. 'Now,' said the producer, 'we are ready. When the green light goes on, begin your talk.' I sat, ready and relaxed, but no green light appeared. The little men ran hither and thither over my library floor, the terrace, the curtilage. 'Finally' the fault was found. The scene was repeated: no green light appeared. After an hour or so of this I diffidently asked, 'I suppose my tape recorder wouldn't do it properly?' Bright smiles flooded the room. The broadcast was made and the van and all the little men and all the apparatus retreated to London.

I never heard my broadcast. I was in an office block in Haymarket with my own family and a number of children belonging to friends. The rain fell steadily. I did not even know that Everest had been. climbed. But a patient a few days later said, 'You needn't deny it, sir. There was me and my 'ubby standing in the rain and suddenly I says to 'im, "Cor, that's the bloody old doctor talkin'." ' This and the cheque is the only evidence I had that it was my voice that announced the success of Hillary and Tenzing on that Coronation morning.

I struggled back rather exhausted from the Haymarket to my house in Chelsea, trying my best to help my wife to deal with what seemed a horde of children. No taxis were available and public transport was so crowded that the thought of getting the children on and off it was unthinkable. We walked. At home a message awaited me. 'Please telephone Lime Grove Studio immediately.' I put the message in the waste-paper basket, poured a pint of beer, lit a pipe, sat down in a comfortable chair and put my feet up on another. Soon the telephone rang (happily within reach) and a peremptory voice asked, 'Didn't you get my message?' 'Yes.' 'Why didn't you ring?' 'I didn't want to.' 'Why not? You didn't know what I wanted.' 'Yes I did.' 'What?' 'You want me on TV.' 'Well, when will you come?' 'I won't. I'm tired.' A long argument followed. Then I said: 'All right: on three conditions.' 'What are they?' 'One – you send a car for me and bring me back.' 'All right. And the next?' 'Double fees.' 'Oh no, that's going too far!' 'All right, I won't come. I don't want to, even for double fees.' Another long argument followed and my demand was agreed. 'Well, you blood-sucker, what's the last?' 'No rehearsal. I'm too tired.' 'Oh, come now, you have really gone too far now.' 'All right, I won't come. I don't want to anyway.' But I won then and nearly lost later. Of course he was right. I sat there with the light upon me (my wife said I looked terribly old) with another camera trained on a series of photographs of Everest and still another on a map. Suddenly I dried up. I had no idea of what I had said or wanted to say. With an extraordinary display of extra-sensory perception the cameras were trained on the photograph and the map. The black-out probably lasted for a few seconds; it seemed minutes to me. It ended and as I began to talk again I was once more on the screen.

But my real story began twenty years earlier.

The Everest Committee looked favourably on our successful ascent of Kamet in 1931 and decided that Smythe, Shipton, Birnie and I should form the nucleus of the 1933 attempt on Everest. Beauman, alas, had not acclimatized well to altitude and Holdsworth could not come.

I had a lot to live up to as the doctor on Everest. Before me had been characters like Tom Longstaff who became President of the Alpine Club and the Royal Geographical Society: like Howard Somervell, a great mountaineer who nearly reached the top, but in addition a painter and musician and the best surgeon on the subcontinent. Then there was Wollaston, a distant family connection, who spent all his life in the pursuit of adventure. He explored not only mountains but also jungles. In New Guinea he was said to have lived with cannibals. Someone asked him how he liked human flesh. 'I never tasted it.' 'Oh, come now, not even a little taste?' 'Well, perhaps I once had a little of the gravy.' The story may be apocryphal: certainly he makes no reference to it in his letters to his wife, but perhaps he wouldn't. He had a sad end. Retiring from adventure to the quiet retreat of King's College, Cambridge, he was murdered by an undergraduate named Potts.

Potts had left Cambridge in the middle of term to live with a prostitute in Jermyn Street taking with him a revolver, for he was a romantic and something of a Walter Mitty. The prostitute, a sensible girl with a proper respect for the proprieties, had persuaded him to return to Cambridge and to apologize to his tutor, Wollaston. It so happened that a police sergeant decided on that day to call on Potts to remind him in the friend-liest way that his fire-arms licence had expired. Being told by the porter that Potts was absent he decided to leave a message with his tutor and was in the middle of doing so when the culprit arrived, misconstrued the presence of the police and shot both Wollaston and the sergeant dead before turning the revolver on himself.

I decided to start the journey by train to Marseille, where I could join a P. & O. ship to Bombay. Trains can be adventurous vehicles. Strange encounters seem always to be about to sway themselves down the long brown corridors, bumping now against the panoramic windows, now flinging themselves uninvited into one's lap. They may be funny, too. There was an earlier time when the members of the Oxford University Mountaineering Club, bound for the mountains of Switzerland, soaked through with the spray of a Channel crossing which had left no complexion untinged, had decided, since the train would not stop before Paris, to strip themselves naked and to dry their clothes by attaching them at regular intervals to a hundred feet of alpine line. The line flung hard from the window, lay along the train, exposing to the startled eyes of travellers in the rear coaches an assortment of undergarments of various materials, sizes and degrees of raggedness. The train, unfortunately, stopped, and not merely deposited the rope, robbed of the horizontal component of its velocity, upon the track, but administered a major shock to the French family which attempted to invade our unclothed privacy. The dignity of the middle-aged and elderly members of the French nation was a subject of general ribaldry in those days. Once on a similar expedition, we had perforce to share the compartment with a family the most noticeable member of which was a black dog, who appeared to be the end product of the casual associations down the years of almost all known breeds. The manners of his many thoroughbred ancestors having thus suffered a gradual dilution, he was prevented by no pride of race from respecting my feet, from which before settling myself to sleep I had removed my heavy climbing boots. As day dawned I discovered his error and flung my socks from the window. Unfortunately we happened to be approaching a small country station, whose master, clad in dignity and much gold braid, received the unsavoury missile on the nose. Unfortunately also, the train again made an unexpected and quite unnecessary halt, apparently for the purpose of allowing the driver, with admirable opportunism, to further his interests with a young girl of pleasing aspect who followed some ill-defined occupation on the line. Only the sudden and apparently unsatisfactory conclusion of this conversation prevented my denouncement to the irate stationmaster by my travelling companions, who, already inflamed against me by my insistence on an open window, openly resented the epithets which I had applied to their faithful friend.

The P. & O. in those days, well supported by the mail contract, cared little for the comfort of its travellers. It was apt to serve the roast beef of Old England, from which the taste had been long removed by unnecessarily adequate refrigeration, whenever the thermometer rose above 90°F. It is curious that whereas the Italians, less conscious perhaps of a sea-going tradition, were prepared to regard their ships as what indeed they are, floating hotels whose one object should be the comfort of their guests, the English at that time continued to regard their liners as parts of a navy barely second to the Royal Navy itself, in which it was an honour to travel. General Charles Bruce used to say that it was a physical effort to him not to stand to attention and salute the captain of a P. & O. liner as he passed his chair on his daily inspection of the ship, dignified, aloof and profoundly contemptuous of the land-lubbers littering his spotless decks. Yet now and again how delightful are the exceptions to this rule, for several times I have travelled in one ship of this very line whose officers were so approachable and so solicitous for one's comfort that not even the Triestino-Lloyd with its exquisite catering could make the journey to India more enjoyable. It was a convenience too, to be able to talk easily with one's steward and have one's desires understood, even if they could not be granted. The barrier which separates an Englishman from a Lascar, still more from a Javanese on a Dutch ship, could be embarrassing, as when, returning from Morocco, I once fell in with a trio of Oxford undergraduates, two men and a girl, who to the amazement and disgust of the Javanese, refused to allow her baggage to be put in any of our cabins and resolutely insisted that she would sleep alone. For hours the little brown men, sitting on their haunches in the passage, chattered their shrill indignation at such wanton waste of good feminine material.

But the decision had been made and the journey begun. No romance or humour enlightened it, till on the midday we reached Marseilles, then a very dirty city, where the streets were full of ordure and garbage, where women washed their linen in the flowing gutters. But as evening fell we ascended in a lift to the summit of the suspension ferry and saw the lights of the city laid out in a gigantic crescent about the harbour, curiously beautiful in the merciful darkness. Alas the lift has gone.

There is no better place than a ship when one is tired of people, tired of adjusting oneself as a doctor must to a rapid succession of other men and women, many sick in body but all in mind. Sometimes as the winter wore on and the panel surgery became more crowded with the coming of February, I thought of myself as the gate-keeper of the Zoological Gardens on a busy afternoon. Click goes the gate (influenza); click (influenza); click (a boil); click (this patient looks ill, there must be something really the matter); click click click (I'm missing all these, make your diagnosis quickly, the crowd is gathering, T.B., acne, gastric ulcer, septic finger, good, I caught up three clicks there). On a ship it is so easy to create a reputation for boorish unsociability that one can be sure of the privacy of a moral leper after the first twenty-four hours. The self-elected sports secretary is easily dealt with. 'Would you like to make a four at deck-tennis, sir?' 'I dislike deck-tennis.' 'Then perhaps you would help me (subtle flattery) to start some other game?' 'I dislike all games.' Sometimes more difficult is the woman (always middle-aged and unsightly) who has found your name in the passenger list and has sought you out because she rather thinks that she once met your cousin John, or dear Mr Higginbotham, who must have been at Oxford at about your time. A fervent denial of any relationship with John or knowledge of Higginbotham is not enough. The only protection is a polite but firm denial of one's own identity, a ruse which cuts the ground from beneath the feet of the most persistent invader of one's privacy. By such devices one can be sure at last of the loneliness which one wants, loneliness to browse upon the ever-changing design of wave and swell; to see the first hint of the cliffs of Corsica on the far horizon; the faint glow in the sky above Stromboli; Sicily, grey and misty in the late afternoon or in early morning pushing first her brick-red hills, then the green slopes, the golden shore above the trout-bright sea.

The ship was in many ways more comfortable than those I had sailed in before. It was decorated, regardless of expense, in a repulsive style, but had a good swimming bath. The food was about what one would expect in one of Joe Lyons' better restaurants, and the company not exciting. We found a soul-mate in one Golding, returning to his post as manager of the Army and Navy Stores in Calcutta. Always immaculate, he attracted the attention of a young officer returning to his Indian unit. One evening as Golding and I leant on the rail in conversation and contemplation of the flying fish, he shyly approached. 'Forgive my impertinence,' he said to Golding, 'but I have so much admired your clothes. Where do you buy them? Do you mind my asking?' 'Not at all, dear boy,' said Golding. 'The Army and Navy Stores, Calcutta.' 'Thank you, Mr Golding. I shall go there as soon as possible.' He strolled on and Golding, putting a hand to his mouth, said, 'Hawes and Curtis, of course.'

At Port Said, Malcolm Pearson came aboard. Malcolm had shared a tutor with me at Oxford. He was, I suppose, one of the most superficially unattractive people I had met. Small, meagre, with an unruly mass of black curly hair, misshapen features and a cockney accent, I shuddered to think of how much time I was fated to spend with him. He became my most intimate friend until his death about twenty years later. Intellectually brilliant, the son of George Pearson who had built the British film industry, he had a fantastic knowledge of art and literature and music. He was a brilliant draftsman who never used his gifts, which were sardonic and witty. He never used any of his gifts. He became a pathologist but not an original one. He drifted through life, enjoying himself in his own sardonic way, completely lacking in the last infirmity of noble minds, finding occupation in the Near and Far East, using his pathological knowledge to earn just sufficient money, of which he needed little.

He passed his examinations with difficulty, though he knew far more than I or any of his contemporaries. His style of dress would not now be a handicap. In those days we went to our viva voce examinations conventionally dressed and tidy. Malcolm's dress was invariably *outré* and his general appearance unkempt and he made no attempt to conform. Finally I took him in hand and brought him to Moss Bros. and to a good hairdresser before his viva: he passed at once. In 1933 he was working as a junior doctor in a scruffy hospital in Port Said. He showed me round and where to buy a topee at Simon Artz which I never wore again. We had many drinks together at the Eastern Exchange Hotel and I was introduced to his latest mistress, a squat person imported from Russia via Shanghai, with whom he was blissfully happy.

Port Said was still a boundary between East and West. Across this boundary for centuries had flowed the religions, commerce and art of the opposing camps. Mahomet had invaded the West and Christ (who, though born an Asiatic Jew, had become an honorary European) the East. The leather and brass of Benares were sold in the Army and Navy Stores and the deficiencies made good by the furnaces of Birmingham. The bead curtains of Araby concealed the intimate nooks of the drawing-rooms of South Kensington and water closets had invaded the private apartments of oriental despots. I had seen turbans on the heads of the ladies of New York and a Homburg hat on that of a Mongolian chief. But still Port Said remained a town without beauty or charm, exercising under the magic sway of Simon Arzt a powerful influence on the minds of men. Here on an Eastern journey the men cast aside their Western hats and bought their Bombay bowlers, and the women remembered with a laugh that was only half a laugh, which had lost a little of the tinkle of the drawing-room and acquired the deeper note of the meadows and groves of Arcadia, that East of Suez the

Ten Commandments do not hold, and for women there is only one significant commandment, even in the West. A change came over the ship. Tropical suits appeared and those men who could trust their legs took to shorts. Arguments began in the evening between those who wore a black coat with white trousers and those who preferred a white coat with black trousers.

The town of Port Said is a place to hear rather than to see. I cannot remember much of its appearance now, but I know that this does not matter. I remember instead the shrill cries of the vendors in their boats selling unwanted things: 'Buy a nice rug, Mrs Langtry,' 'You throw me sixpence, Mr Ramsay Macdonald,' 'Hi, Mr Lloyd George, look you, only five pounds,' all spoken with the suggestion of a Glasgow accent beneath their Egyptian intonation. Any of these, when asked his name would give a Scottish one in reply, yet his unequivocal blackness denied the suggestion of mixed parentage. The guides had the memories of Oxford scouts, one, whose name was Macpherson, remembering me embarrassingly as the member of a party which had had curious adventures in his company years before. From that moment of recognition we were besieged and greeted by name by all the riff-raff of Port Said, who attempted unsuccessfully to drag us, midday though it was, to every haunt of vice the town could provide, offering us their nearest and dearest relations with touching testimonials and descriptions of their skill which left nothing to the most perverted imagination. From the deepest slums of the town came sellers of every worthless thing from collar studs to 'feelthy pictures', the last and most adhesive of whom was only dismissed by my solemn statement that I had taken his photographs myself with my own camera. It was this very man who had on a previous journey sold his finest collection at a shocking price to a naval officer and palmed off on him instead two dozen identical photographs of the Eastern Exchange Hotel, a fact which he only discovered when he later spread them for the delight of his friends upon the smoking-room table.

The journey down the Suez Canal can be very pleasant in February. Later, in May, the sunbaked shores begin to produce those confusing moving shapes which have given to the eastern side its name of the Country of the Mirage. As one sat on deck, looking out across that vast expanse of sand, features began to appear, hills and little woods and shaded expanses of water, trembling in the haze of heat. One had been warned. That, one said, is a mirage. Yet as one approached the trembling became less, the outline firmer, and a real hill sailed by on the port side. The curious black smudge must indeed have been real, though one could not see quite what it was. It too came nearer, clearer, and suddenly became a clump of palms and a moment later disappeared, melting into the shimmering haze of sand. There was no criterion of reality by which one might judge these scenes for true or false.

We passed Sinai by night and in the morning lay beneath its huge red cliffs. Then all day we saw no land until the sun went down behind the tiny distant peaks of Africa, leaving behind it an aquamarine sky, stripped with hard lines of black and gold beneath a purple cirrhus dappled with orange light.

An Egyptian prince with a hennaed Frenchwoman too strongly perfumed had appeared at Port Said. Tonight as he entered the smoking-room four serious Americans rose and bowed but saw us smiling and hurriedly sat down. We had entered the tropics. I stood in the bows with the warm damp south wind in my face. The sky was very bright with stars which, as one's eye approached the southern horizon had about them a strangely foreign look. The sea was bright with darting masses of phosphorescent spray, like meteors in the foam of our passage. A real shooting star shot suddenly across the sky. Perhaps, I thought, it is sometimes better not to be alone. The elderly astronomer at my side continued to expound the recession of the spiral nebulae.

It was raining in Aden, an almost unheard of event. The Americans went ashore to see the stuffed mermaids and returned disappointed and disconsolate. The Indian Ocean was oily and calm. After four days of its unchanging surface, the vulgar occidentalism of Bombay came as a relief to the monotony.

In Bombay the Englishman of those days came into his own. Surrounded by a race which admitted its inferiority by a slavish deference varied only and rarely by a feeble and ill-directed violence he sloughed the shyness which had hitherto imprisoned him. Beyond the vast Victorian pseudo-oriental portals of the Gateway of India he was the Master. A match for the average Indian in physique, in cunning and even often in intelligence, he knew that even in death he was paramount, slain because he was the Master, dying at the hand of slaves. He found this a pleasant and encouraging thought. The Gateway of India for him was a gateway to self-confidence, and when in the fullness of time he retired to Bath or Oxford or Cheltenham he took with him a model of the gateway in ivory or brass to remind him that once he was a Man.

But to me, though not in my deepest heart immune from such thoughts, Bombay was the city not of the Gateway, nor even of the long bar of the Taj Mahal Hotel, but the city of dark and hideous alleys, of streets where unlovely girls sat for sale behind iron bars in Grant Road.

The study of houses of ill-fame is full of interest to the curious, and often in no way unpleasant. At Muleh Abdulla, in the Arab quarter of Fez, every house is open. In a pleasant courtyard under a fig tree Jim and I were served with coffee by a girl who showed in dress and manner nothing of her profession save for this – she was unveiled. In this stronghold of the Faith no alcohol was, of course, allowed, and there was thus absent from the atmosphere that indecorum which not even the most fervent supporter of wine can deny that it brings in its train. No advertising of the wares in this emporium occurred, no pressing of unwilling customers. Only now and again a man would cease to play upon his guitar (for most of the customers brought their instruments for the entertainment of the rest) and would discreetly withdraw with the girl and her coffee. Only one incident marred the decorous scene. A French taxi-driver, drunk and therefore shocking already in all eyes, came singing loud and ribald songs and adopted towards a serving girl a disrespectful manner, like that which her French counterpart would doubtless expect. Two dignified and bearded men approached and with polite bows made gentle remonstrance. He laughed in their faces. Still polite, each took him by an elbow and, lifting him effortlessly, carried him out, his legs kicking vainly in the air. When a minute later they returned, still grave and impassive, they were flicking from their robes a few drops of water from the nearby fountain.

At Bombay my old Kamet servant Lall came aboard. How he knew I was there I never discovered for his English was as bad as my Pushtu. But there he was, having travelled by what means I do not know from his home somewhere in the north-west, ready with a wreath of flowers to put round my neck, confident that I would need him again. Bonham, an old friend, was there to smooth our passage with his usual efficiency and the usual flow of beer. We walked to the Taj Mahal Hotel. 'How *was* the Taj Mahal?' said Frank Smythe for the hundredth time. 'Unbelievable,' I obediently replied. The band played all the tunes to which I had so recently danced with the main reason that had nearly prevented my journey: 'We just couldn't say goodbye,' 'Say it isn't so', 'Night and Day'. I became rather dreamy over my beer, wondering whether I was doing the right thing, whether I wanted to be so far from Quaglino's. I *was* doing the right thing. In the ensuing months I at last made up my mind and made it up aright.

All next day we ran across the dull Indian plains, the view occasionally broken by long tree-covered escarpments, stopping often at small, ugly, evil-smelling stations. There had been rain, unusual in February, and the ricefields were bright apple-green, and the whole countryside more coloured than I had seen it before. In the afternoon a hailstorm broke, stones the size of hazelnuts rattling on the coach and bouncing off the platforms, beating down the mauve and purple bougainvillaea on the station walls. At sunset, inky black clouds hung in great masses over a dark orange sky. Flashes of lightning illuminated trees swaying in the wind on the horizon. Crashes of thunder drowned the noise of the loudest train on earth.

Calcutta was full of parties. I stayed with Wilfred Hunter and his lovely wife, getting to bed in the not-so-small hours and breakfasting on the lawn, surrounded by dahlias and buddleias and the calling of birds, the homely caw of rooks, the monotonous tapping of the brain-fever bird, the loud yell of a big black unknown fowl and the high gargle of another. But there was much to do, testing oxygen apparatus and reviewing stores before we left for Darjeeling.

Of Darjeeling I remember little except the daybreak of the first day when I was awakened by Ferdie Crawford's cry of 'Come out on to the balcony, you clot.' I could see nothing but thick mist, swishing downwards into an invisible valley. Ferdie put a firm hand under my chin and pushed back my head. Above the misty horizon, Kanchenjunga, only apparently a mile or two away, lay in the brilliant light of early morning, the snow tinged with a golden light, the combes in deep shadow, the vast mass of the mountain seeming about to fall on the defenceless town. Everybody has heard of the view of Everest from Tiger Hill – a little unimportant knob that no one would notice were it not the highest mountain in the world. But the view of Kanchenjunga is unforgettable.

From Darjeeling the road winds in a quick series of almost unbelievable bends downwards to the plains and into the jungle of the Terai. In a clearing at Sukna lived Mrs Wrangham-Hardy's cow elephant, a lovely animal who, having been wounded in the lists of love by a wild gallant from the forest, had developed an abscess on the spine of which she was likely to die. I do not know why a physician should have been chosen, as there was in those days in Darjeeling a highly skilled surgeon, but I was persuaded to operate upon this animal. I took with me the largest knife I could find in the kitchen of the Planters' Club, a length of rubber hose from the garden, a tablespoon sharpened on the dusty road below the quarter-deck of the Club and some tarred string.

I was nervous of my reception and my fears were realized. The designers of anaesthetic masks (and every anaesthetist worthy of the name has designed at least one) have entirely forgotten to fit one for the trunk of an elephant. In Darjeeling I was unable to find a hypodermic needle capable of piercing the hide of a pachyderm. So anaesthesia was impossible. The

123

elephant not unnaturally resented the first cut and, rising hurriedly to her feet, set out to look for the surgeon, who by that time was hidden behind a tree. The mahouts persuaded her again to lie still, but the second cut produced a still more cataclysmic heaving and my still more rapid retreat. The cleaning out of the cavity of the abscess, which was proportional to the elephant and about the size of a Rugby football, she bore stoically and even the sewing in of the hose with a sadler's needle and tarred string produced only a minor earthquake. The dangerous work done, the owner and I sat at the edge of the clearing and had tea. It was then that there appeared out of the forest a very beautiful peacock whom I rather unwisely fed with a cheese biscuit. The result was most unexpected. The bird emitted a series of such appalling screams that I feared he must be allergic to cheese and would soon expire horribly. It soon appeared, however, that the cacophony was caused by a strong desire for more. The great bird's addiction to cheese and consequent cupboard love for me became such a nuisance that we gathered up our belongings and, accompanied by our tormentor, who, guessing our object, was now making the forest hideous with sound, made for the car. Amidst a crescendo of wails which drowned the sound of the self-starter we left. A mile or two away from the clearing I looked behind. Along the very middle of the road, dusty and drab, tottering now with fatigue but sticking to his monomaniac quest, was the peacock. The way began its tortuous climb towards Darjeeling and in its turns the fond bird was lost to view.

After a few delightful days in Kalimpong the journey to Everest really began. The way led partly along a high dusty path, partly along open hillside through orchards in blossom, partly through light jungle in which the insects, bent on sexual pleasures, made a noise like a thousand self-starters. Then, after Pedong, it lay through thick and airless jungle to a glorious bathe in the Rongpo river on the border of India and Sikkim. For the first time in my life I owned a horse, a Bhutia whom I called April 5th, after a horse I once backed in the Derby. The horse had won but the bookmaker had welshed: this was my revenge. On April 5th I rode through dense forest to the bungalow at Pakhyong and a view of many miles of the dense forest of Sikkim.

Next day, more jungle paths led to Gangtok, capital of Sikkim, a clean and colourful village. Here we were received by His Highness the Maharajah, a small, shy and ineffectual individual. Perhaps it was as well for him that he was so, for his father and elder brother (once of my college, Pembroke, where, in that nest of singing birds as Samuel Johnson called it, he had acquired a dangerous individuality of song), had both been poisoned by the lamas, who had found it unnecessary to murder the present king. The year before they had foretold his death, a touchy moment. No one seemed to know how he had erred, but he must have seen the error of his ways for the lamas, by urgent prayer, had saved his life. The chief lama, known as Rimpoche, appeared to be something of a Rasputin. He was said to be the Maharajah's elder half brother, having been born on his mother's long journey with the Sikkimese equivalent of Tristan from Lhasa to Gangtok, to her wedding with his father. Such incidents were regarded as inevitable on such journeys, owing to the coldness of the nights, and were no obstacle to the ensuing festivities. Fortunately for the present sovereign, his young and beautiful wife shared her mother-in-law's predilection for lamas and periodically went into diplomatic retreat for purposes it was rumoured, of prayer and fasting. Her offspring were certainly a credit to the religious life and large for so small a father. For a reason we never discovered she had spent the night before our arrival at the dak bungalow where we stayed and had left her tiny shoes under our leader's bed. We were sorry her arrival and departure had been so premature.

One of the inexplicable things about the mysterious East is the deterioration in taste with time. Countries like China, India, Japan, that have in the past produced objects of great loveliness, now mix the old and beautiful with the new and hideous with all the effrontery of an Oxford don, capable of allowing so offensive a building as Mr Maxwell's book and record ship to defile the view of Magdalen and its bridge, one of the loveliest in

Europe. Here in Gangtok the beautiful temple was locked by an object in black japan characteristic of the Victorian kitchen quarters. The king's palace was like a cheap hotel in an unfashionable English seaside resort. His Highness came to lunch with us wearing over an orange silk shirt a long robe of royal blue brocade – but on his head was a little tweed hat and on his feet shoes that were too yellow and too pointed, straight from the East End of London.

The charms of Gangtok were too much for our porters and we started late for Karponang. Up a good wide path we walked through a forest of rhododendron and magnolia till the way opened up to disclose a carpet of primula, potentilla, gentian and ranunculus. Occasional drifts of snow occurred and a cold wind began to blow.

Every morning we were awakened by the cheerful shouts of Shebbeare, our transport officer, who awoke at five-thirty whatever the time arranged for breakfast. The upgetting of the 'she bear sahib' was the signal to the porters to bring us our morning tea. By six the ringing of bells announced the arrival of the mules and by six-thirty our servants were trying to steal the beds from beneath our still dozing bodies. From Karponang we had a pleasant ten-mile walk up a steadily climbing track. The magnolia were now far below us and the forest was of juniper and rhododendron, the floor still thickly strewn with primulas growing between patches of snow. At about 11,000 feet, the primulas grew scanter and silver fir gradually supplanted the juniper. The great rhododendron trees gave place to a smaller bushier shrub like that of England but gentians still edged the path. The path hairpinned its way up a long valley where snow lay thick. At 12,000 feet a few flakes began to fall and we rounded a corner to the lake of Tsongo, a frozen stretch of water a half-mile broad, beyond which lay our bungalow. Here I removed an upper molar tooth from my servant Passang Tentsing, the second dental operation since student days.

We rose early on a morning of crisp snow and a cloudless sky. By ten-thirty we were on the summit of the Natu La, where was a vast cairn ornamented with prayer flags to which our porters added theirs. Beyond the cairn Chomolhari lay clear against the horizon, a perfect triangle of rock and snow. An easy track led us downhill through a forest of silver pine and juniper, the snow-free patches blue with gentian, to the bungalow of Chumbitang. In the evening Hugo Boustead and I climbed a little hill and saw Chomolhari change from black and white to autumn brown and pink in the setting sun, lying above a long bank of pale grey cloud, seemingly impossible high above the brown Tibetan hills. The glow faded, leaving the great triangle a pale grey against an ink-blue sky.

We were in Tibet.

11 Through Tibet to Everest

At seven-thirty we set out on the easy downhill twelve-mile walk to Yatung, through silver pines and junipers and primulas and white everlasting flowers. Down at 11,000 feet roses and spiraeas grew amidst blue pines. We came upon a monastery round which we were shown by the artist called down from Lhasa to redecorate its walls with paintings more decorous than those they replaced. The track below was infested with red ticks, which worried me somewhat, and festooned with prayer flags, perhaps as a protection against typhus: if so they were very successful. In a small village through which we passed a murderer lay on his blanket in the muddy street, unable to find shelter in any house. He had received a hundred and fifty lashes, for there was no death penalty in Tibet, where life was sacred. I dressed his wounds and sent him some food and felt glad to live in a country that at that time knew the mercy of capital punishment. A suspected murderer in Tibet was beaten on alternate days with a hide whip until he confessed, in which case he had another final beating. He was then handed over to the beggars whose responsibility it was to see that he did not starve. Punishment for theft varied according to the seriousness of the offence from the loss of an ear to the loss of one or both hands or feet. There was almost no crime in Tibet.

So into the Chumbi Valley, with its memories of Younghusband's expedition of thirty years before. There was still a platoon there of British soldiers. We galloped across the old battlefield, passed several frozen waterfalls like organ pipes of pale green ice and came to the bungalow of Gaotsa and our advance party awaiting us.

Soon the country changed. Signs of human habitation were no longer to be seen. We walked into a wide glacier valley of light snow surrounded by brown rolling hills, a waste trackless but for the single telegraph wire from India to Lhasa, strangely out of place in that primaeval wilderness. Though I had taken to my pony and cantered much of the way we seemed hardly to move in the vast featureless landscape until suddenly two miles away we saw the fort of Phari, lying beneath the huge triangle of Chomolhari, rose pink where the precipice was too steep for the snow to lie.

The fort, or dzong, lay in the centre of a village reputed to be the dirtiest in Asia. The houses, of one storey only, were built of rough unmortared stone and were roofed with rotting turf. The sewage was discharged directly into the streets, if the narrow muddy evil-smelling alleys between the houses could be dignified by such a word. It was impossible to walk a few yards without traversing a dung heap. The skins and clothes of the people were black with the dirt of ages. They crowded round our camp fire with horribly adjacent curiosity or sat staring on the nearer dung-hills. Their filthy pariah dogs, less trustful than their human counterparts, surrounded the outskirts of our compound and howled dismally through the night. A mile or two to the north the perfect outline and pure cleanliness of Chomolhari made a heartless contrast to the city built on dung.

It was on the next day, a morning of warm sun and cloudless sky, that we became acquainted with the so-called afternoon wind of Tibet. It begins to blow at dawn and continues until nightfall, blowing into one's eyes, nose, ears and mouth a mixture of fine red dust and the dried excrement of a thousand years of travellers across the high plateau. Tom Brocklebank, Jack Longland, George Wood-Johnson and I explored the abominable little town, picking our way through the ordure to the dzong, outwardly an architectural triumph of great dignity set upon a high rock, inwardly in keeping with its filthy setting. From the flat roof one could see the little houses of Phari bright with prayer flags and half a mile away the monastery set on a twin hill. Beyond in all directions stretched the brown Tibetan plain, now almost free from snow. Beyond again were brown hills streaked with snow and, overtopping them, range after range of peaks, Chomolhari, the mountains of Bhutan, Kanchenjunga and Pauhunri, white and jagged against a deep blue sky.

I took my horse and rode up to a neighbouring col beyond which lay Bhutan. Returning down the rough mountainside I saw ahead of me the angle between two brown hillsides sub-tending the distant ranges turning from white to steely grey in the failing light; saw below them the plain of Phari turn from brown to a deeper grey, zoned with the purple shadows of approaching snow clouds; saw at last the monastery, a black cone against a plain from which all colour had now gone. April 5th stumbled on in the darkness towards the line of tents below the dzong, which looked now like Edinburgh Castle, tripping into pica holes and shying at snow patches, an idiot horse but my own. In my tent a great contentment surrounded me for the first time since Kamet. I wrote in my diary 'Tents are better than houses, oh, so much better'.

We rode on next day, in a rather feeble attempt at a blizzard, encountering every few minutes a train of mules or yaks with richly embroidered saddlery and tinkling bells. When the way steepened I handed April 5th to a seis and Frank Smythe and I walked together, finding that at 15,000 feet we could go as effortlessly as on an English moor. Acclimatization to altitude was progressing well. After three hours we came to the Tang La and saw before us an illimitable yellow plain streaked with snow, in the middle of which we pitched camp in a strong wind. The temperature fell during the afternoon and the wind blew more strongly but we sat warm and comfortable in the mess tent until at five o'clock Ferdie Crawford called us out.

Above us were the gigantic cliffs of Chomolhari, snow hanging precariously to its less precipitous slopes, elsewhere red against a sky of cloudless blue, save where a whisp of cloud trailed like lawn from the mountain-top. In all other directions the white and yellow plain stretched far away, flat as a calm sea, to blue rocky peaks low on the horizon. The sun was setting behind a bank of cloud and its last rays made a pale golden path across the plain, sometimes sparkling on the snow, sometimes merging with the sand.

That night the temperature fell to —2°F, 34 degrees of frost. In the morning we cantered and trotted across level frozen snow. The sky remained clear but a mighty wind blew the snow in our faces. The snow began to melt and going became difficult for the horses. We dismounted and led them protesting along a track we could no longer see.

It was on this day and in these meteorological circumstances, that the transport arrangements broke down. The mess tent, which should have been ahead of us, had been overtaken and we could expect no hot meal to welcome us at our next camping place. Indeed no one seemed to know where this would be. Wood-Johnson, whose responsibility this was, had disappeared. We came to a ridge that fell away steeply into another yellow snow-streaked plain and with difficulty persuaded our horses to descend. As no one else seemed inclined to take the responsibility in Wood-Johnson's absence, I found a good camping site high in a yellow valley below the Donkya La and set off at a gallop to find the mess tent and kitchen, which I located some two miles away, but of our personal porters there was no sign. Gradually through the afternoon they drifted in, having found the snow as much as they could bear. I took a wicked pleasure in the talk of my companions, who considered that they had had a hell of a day. I had greatly enjoyed it.

All next day the sun shone and, though the 'afternoon wind' got up at about ten o'clock, it was never strong or cold enough to bother us. We walked and rode over country like the South Downs of England, but yellow, not green, and without vegetation of any kind. We crossed three passes, each time dipping down into yellow valleys between high yellow cliffs. The next day's march was, in the words of *The Fight for Everest*, 'across a dreary and desolate plain'. The temperature was 10°F. But the sun shone and the sky was cloudless. There were occasional cushions of flowers which would soon make the plain a thing of beauty. Kanchenjunga and the Jonsong peak were visible in the distance, balanced on a layer of mirage. Low rolling yellow hills obscured much of the distant view, but far ahead we could see the great dark blue peaks lying above the Brahmaputra, falling away towards us in yellow downs. After two hours of walking Smijth-Windham, Wood-Johnson and I sat down beneath a great cliff, sheltered from the cold wind and basked for an hour in brilliant sunshine. An hour later we rode into camp, pitched ready for us beneath a conical rock surmounted by a nunnery.

It was a small windowless building. It was dark and very dirty, smelling of human sweat and excreta and burning rancid butter. On the walls, filthy, torn and untended, hung thankgas of great loveliness. The nuns, some fifteen in number, varied in age from young girls to aged crones, and were clad in black habits that had once been red. They were adorned with huge wigs of black wool that had once been green, showing their original colour near the scalp and reminding me of the heads of western demi-blondaines whose dyed yellow locks had failed to conceal the original brown of their hair.

We left not unwillingly next day. Ferdie Crawford and I rode over a slight rise into yet another great yellow plain, fringed on the left by the great distant peaks of Pauhunri, Kanchenjunga and Chomolhari. On the hillside above herds of gazelle and wild asses grazed on apparently non-existent grass. A hare with green fur dashed suddenly across our path and two orioles came fearlessly to investigate our chocolate papers. This was more colourful country. The yellow of the desert was relieved by banks of purple across the hillsides and occasional meadows of coarse, pale green tufted grass. We crossed a pass of 17,500 feet and descended into a broad valley in which a stream ran. It narrowed into a winding gorge, then opened into a great basin. On our left a yellow cliff was crowned by a great cream fortress that continued in its walls the backward slant of the rock on which it stood, seeming to be a part of its own natural foundations. Beyond lay our green tents and beyond them, cut out in white and dark blue cardboard between desert and sky, were the greater Himalaya.

Here, at Khamba Dzong, we spent three days. The place was

beautifully warm and sunny but afflicted by the ubiquitous filthy dust of Tibet, so that sore throats affected many of us, porters and sahibs alike. We were shown the fort by the Niapala, his chief the Dzong Pen himself being in Lhasa, receiving the high Tibetan title of Dzaza. On the roof were several slate bas-reliefs of Buddhist deities, exquisitely carved, lying broken in odd corners. In the library, a dark and dirty room with small paper windows, shelves of books lay decaying deep in dust. If Curzon's Levantine loot and Elgin's Greek purchases were justified, here would be an equally justifiable theft. But the Tibetans are just enough sophisticated to protect their treasures from foreigners, though not from dirt and decay.

We made a pilgrimage to the grave of Dr Kellas, who died here in 1921. Fragments only of the inscription survived. We hauled into position a stone that we hoped was too large for the villagers to break and while Shebbeare read Psalm 121 I tried to carve a fresh inscription. The stone was too hard and my tools too blunt, but the lamas promised to complete the task in return for three rupees. I have never heard whether they succeeded. Whether or not they completed the inscription it is certain that no doctor has a lovelier resting place.

Hugh Ruttledge and I rode out of Khamba discussing plans for our assault on the mountain. Already the party, on the grounds of character, physical fitness and climbing ability was beginning to sort itself out into three categories and we were able even at this early stage tentatively to assign their later functions. April 5th was going badly. For some days he had been off his feed and losing weight. His coat seemed loose and was no longer glossy. We overtook the yak column and lay and rested in the shelter of a ruined village and watched the antics of a grey and cream lizard some four inches long (*pythrocephalus theobaldi*). April 5th found it difficult to rise and I walked on, leading him unburdened by any load. The wind got up, not very cold but very strong in our faces. For mile after mile we pushed on, leading the sick horse towards the little distant hamlet of Lingga. The dust swept towards us in yellow clouds that cut out the view and made us bow our heads in an unsuccessful attempt to protect our eyes, or revolved in great columns across the desert floor. In Lingga we were again ahead of the transport but our long wait was enlivened by a visit from three pretty Tibetan girls with warm brown skins, high cheekbones and slanting Mongol eyes. I had already conducted my customary out-patient session, which made us disinclined for closer contact with them. Here I exchanged horses with Frank, who disliked riding. Forbra, whom I took in exchange, was a white horse with a tendency to be skittish but the most comfortable amble and canter one could wish for. Frank was terrified of him and much happier leading April 5th who from then on lived a life of slothful ease and gradually recovered.

After Lingga the plain became more colourful, covered with coarse green grass. From ten miles away we could see Tengkye Djong. It was warm and sunny and there was no wind. The plain ended in a cirque of low hills set with little villages, ancient forts and white monasteries, an important centre of population.

The dzong lay white in the afternoon sun beyond a great lake on which Brahmini ducks swam solemnly, not speaking to the Barheads. It was a huge rectangular building with a flat roof and the usual Tibetan concourse of lesser houses leaning against it for support. Inside it was a maze of little galleried courtyards and twisting broken stairways and tiny dusty rooms from which peered dog faces, cow faces, human faces. The human faces were as brown and indifferent as the cow faces.

In one little room, less dirty than most, the dzongpen and his wife received us with all the ceremony of palaces. A heap of rugs and skins, on which we sat cross-legged, lay along two sides of the room, which was dimly lit by small paper windows. Several ancient fire-arms and a whip or two decorated the red walls. In one corner a sideboard bore a dozen or so of silver charm boxes studded with turquoise. The ceiling, blackened by an iron stove occasionally refreshed with yak dung, was supported by a carved wooden pillar to which were attached several pages from an ancient issue of the *Illustrated Sporting and Dramatic News*.

The dzongpen was a large man with an amused face and a

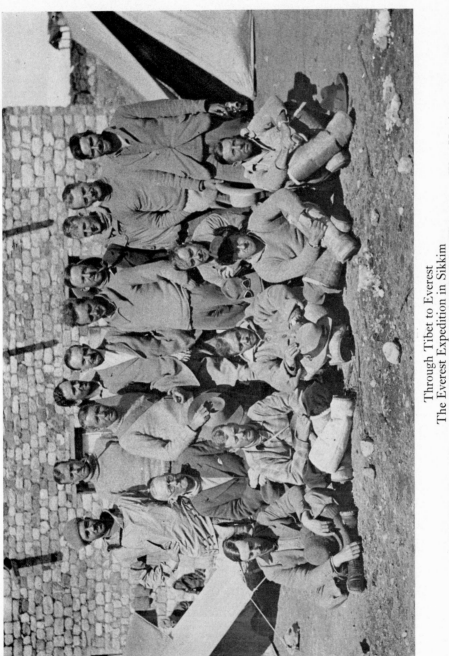

Through Tibet to Everest
The Everest Expedition in Sikkim
Smijth-Windham, Greene, Brocklebank, McLean, Smythe, Thompson, Wyn-Harris
Wood-Johnson, The Political Agent, Shipton
Ruttledge
Longland, Birnie, Wager, Crawford, Boustead
Shebbeare

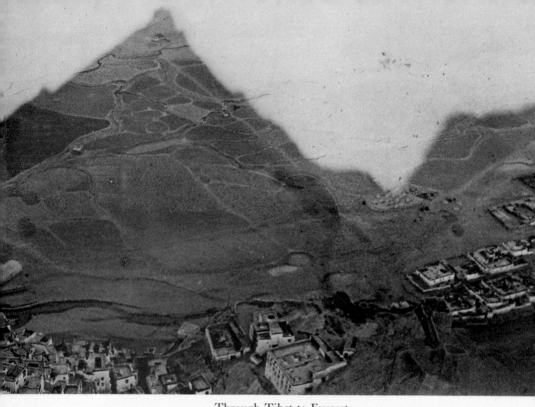

Through Tibet to Everest
View from the summit of Shekar Dzong. The shadow of the hill at sunset

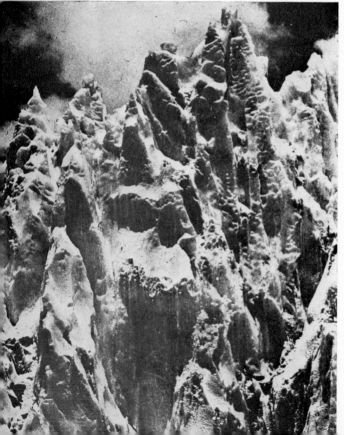

The Everest Adventure
Seracs between Camps I and II
'designed by a megalomaniac
Lalique'

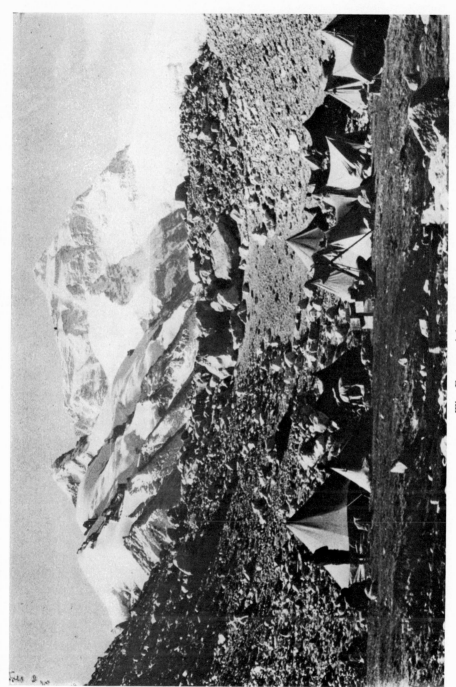

The Everest Adventure
Mount Everest from Base Camp

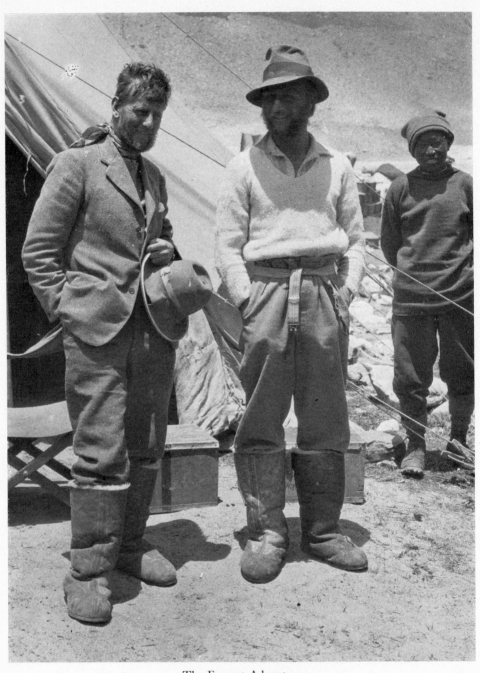

The Everest Adventure
Frank Smythe and Eric Shipton

rather unsuccessful fringe of black beard. His clothes were of great beauty. He wore a long purple brocade robe, black velvet top boots and a fur hat decorated with turquoise and ruby. His wife was a short and fat and smiling and as full of character as a cockney flower woman. She was dressed like any other Tibetan woman, but her great head-dress was elaborately decorated with coral and her charm box gleamed with rubies. Out of our limited wardrobe we had found it impossible to compete, all save Hugh Ruttledge who had succeeded in buying a brown brocade Tibetan overcoat, above which he sported an opera hat which he reserved for state occasions like this.

We sat upon the rugs. On a low divan across the room our servants sat, silent with the natural breeding of the Mongol. Kharma Paul interpreted a long exchange of compliments. Tibetan tea in fine china cups on high silver saucers were put before us. These must be filled three times before a helping may be refused but happily it is not necessary to take more than a sip at a time. A plate of sweets was brought, pleasant crisp biscuits, dried apricots and barley sugar. Then chang appeared, a mildly alcoholic brew from fermented barley, and this we consumed for the rest of the day.

After conversation, music. Three girls appeared, taller and prettier than most Tibetans, with soft caressing speaking voices; they made a most raucous noise when they sang. They sang that in a dream they stood on the summit of Chomolungma and that with them stood a young man (who was George) and an old man like God (who was Hugh) and another old man who was the friend of God (Shebbeare) and a young man who was like the thunderbolt of God (myself). All seven, they said, then drank much chang and became drunk so that they dreamed no more. This seemed to us to be a good omen.

Then a man played on a guitar and the girls danced a simple tap dance, and they brought more chang. The evening began to fade. Outside there was a tinkle of bells and we moved into a gallery surrounding a central court like an English coaching inn. The unshod mules from Sola Khombu stole silently into the yard below us, their scarlet trappings dimmed in the dying light. In their red and green boots the muleteers moved silently among them, the silence broken only by the occasional clear note of a bell.

In the living-room of the fort there was now almost total darkness. The voices of the girls were soft again. They brought more chang.

A long march to Khengu followed this interlude, then a short one to Chiblung. It was here that the accident already described nearly robbed us of our interpreter Karma Paul and our postman Lobsang Tsering, but happily they escaped, the one with a broken little finger and the other with a broken collar bone. Our next march, dusty but not unpleasant, finished down a steep sand-dune falling to the bank of a broad shallow river across which, jumping from island to island, meandered a remarkable bridge constructed of twisted yak hair and odd pieces of timber. We camped in a horseshoe of steep sand in a spot we hoped was protected from the wind from all directions, but the wind came from all directions, including, it seemed from the earth below and heaven above, and filled our tents with dust. On the next day I rode on Forbra across a wide shallow frozen river. Tom Brocklebank crossed without incident ahead of me but must have cracked the ice. When Forbra's front feet were almost on the farther shore he slid back suddenly and began to panic. Realizing that he was in a quicksand, I swung my right leg over his neck, stood up in my left stirrup and, holding the bridle, jumped for the shore. Unfortunately our harness consisted for the most part of cardboard masquerading as leather and tied together with string. Forbra had long since lost his chin strap, so when I pulled the whole harness came off and left me helpless. He slipped back another yard from shore and another two feet deeper into the mud, gave up the struggle and passively began to sink. Luckily at this point two Tibetans appeared on the far shore and by throwing stones and shouting execrations so infuriated him that with a convulsive movement he freed himself and floundered out. He was very wet and cold, so Tom and I raced the last two miles to Trangso Chumbab. Tom on Easter Hero won by a length the first Tibetan Derby.

We planned after this an easy day, but it was not to be. I had no reins and Forbra celebrated his release by being more than usually disobedient. The wind blew steadily and dust filled every natural orifice. It was a curious stretch of country, apparently flat but with an eerie capacity to lose from sight all human occupants. Frank Smythe and I knew that the transport yaks were not far behind and our companions not more than an hour ahead, but for twenty miles we rode on in the teeth of the wind without a sight of human kind. Only the occasional mark of a nailed boot in the dust assured us that we were not lost. We passed a splendid camp site, well sheltered by a pleasant stream, continued for a few more miles, and came to a filthy village called Kishiyong in the middle of which the mess tent had been pitched. Usually my decision about camping sites went unquestioned, but on this occasion my protests were in vain. They only slightly stirred the lethargy of my tired companions: we stayed.

We left on a lovely morning. The wind had dropped and the dust ceased to trouble us. Shekar Dzong was twenty miles ahead and Hugh Ruttledge had promised that we would camp three miles from the town, where smallpox was said to be raging. Bill Birnie and I waited to see the transport away. I made a new harness out of rope and after five miles of easy riding we came to a ramshackle bridge beyond which lay a vast plain. Beyond it was a great conical hill studied with diamonds glistening in the sunshine, the hill of Shekar Dzong.

Of all the places I had seen, Shekar most resembled, from a distance, the fairy palace of my childish dreams. Crowning the hill were the brown ruins of an ancient fort and straggling downwards a hundred white hermits' cells. Nearer the foot lay a gigantic white monastery, clinging precariously to the cliff face, ready at any moment to slide on to the plain below. But the sight that caught my eye as I approached and almost blinded my infuriated gaze to the beauty above was the green mess tent, surrounded by the usual huddle of packing cases and sacks, so close to the edge of the town below the monastery that no picketing could prevent the closest contact with the curious villagers, surrounded by the accumulated filth of an oriental bazaar, its water supply polluted by the fairy-like but obviously insanitary buildings on the hill above, where the black openings of huge elementary wooden drains were connected by long green algal trails with the plain below. Sickened by the sight of such ineptitude I stated firmly but kindly my complete refusal of all responsibility, kindly because Hugh already had enough to worry him.

At some point on the route from Kishiyong wholesale thefts had been committed. The loss of equipment was serious. Porters' altitude boots and clothing, food and alcoholic drink had disappeared. As no one knew exactly when or where the crime had been committed it was impossible definitely to fix the blame on any set of muleteers, whose personnel changed repeatedly. However the discovery of a wet piece of turf where his boots should have been suggested to the logical mind of Lewa the Sirdar that the theft was recent. With a yell of fury he hurled himself on a terrified muleteer, kicked him where it hurt him most and ran him protesting into the presence of the dzongpen.

The dzongpen or commander of the dzong or fort was a small and inconspicuous person in the yellow hat of the fourth rank. He was very anxious to be helpful. He arrested four muleteers and ordered a trial for the afternoon. The complainants were represented of necessity by our leader, and by myself, chosen by the others because something unpleasant was foreseen and it was considered by all (but for a minority of one) that my medical experience best fitted me to withstand whatever was in store.

For half an hour we sat on cushions, drank tea and made polite conversation. No details of the theft were requested. The four ragged suspects were then brought in and warned that unless they confessed their own guilt or told us the names of the guilty they would be whipped. Falling on their knees, weeping loudly, rubbing their noses in the dust, they protested both their innocence and their ignorance.

I had gone to the ceremony expecting to be shocked by the brutality of Tibetan 'justice'. Evidence against these men was completely lacking and I knew that whatever they might say they would be tortured. If they confessed they would be whipped in punishment. If they did not confess, they would be whipped in the hope of extracting information. In fact I was somewhat shocked at myself for not being shocked. Perhaps many weeks in Tibet had begun a process of mental assimilation, an acceptance of the world around me. Perhaps too my heart was a little hardened by what seemed to me a note of insincerity in the wailing that assailed our ears and failed to gain our sympathy. Perhaps I was too disgusted that men should behave with so little dignity or fortitude. For whatever cause I felt no pity for the muleteers and knew that my face was as impassive as the calm Mongolian countenance beside me.

After the men had been given every opportunity to speak, they were removed to the courtyard and we were escorted with much ceremony to the roof. Again the men were given an opportunity to speak but they continued only to wail for mercy. The first man was laid prone upon the ground, his buttocks bared and his wrists and ankles bound. One man held the thong binding his wrists and another the one binding his ankles. By leaning backwards they could keep him nicely on the stretch.

I began to wonder whether I was going to be sick. Instead I drank tea.

A man with a long rawhide whip stood on each side of the muleteer's prostrate form, and, alternately from left and right, the lash fell across his brown skin. Monotonously his wails blended with the monotonous chanting of his executioners numbering the strokes. White weals bisected the brown buttocks, spread, coalesced, till all the skin was white. Then slowly, lazily, the blood began to ooze as each new stroke fell. No reflex contraction of the muscles suggested the agony I knew he must feel. He did not shriek as I thought he would. He continued to wail just as he had wailed before. After fifty strokes he was given another opportunity to speak. He said nothing and was given fifty more. He was then declared innocent and returned to his cell – for who but an innocent man could be so gifted by the Gods with a shut mouth?

To the Westerner the process sounds brutal and unjust and so it was. But there is another side. At the expense of ten minutes of pain, which he obviously did not regard as unbearable, the muleteers of Tibet, amongst whom the news undoubtedly spread fast, had been taught a salutary lesson. The foreigner brought much money to Tibet and should therefore be protected from brigandage. In Sicily fifty years ago to rob a foreigner was punished by the Mafia with death.

I did not wait to see the beating of the other three muleteers. I had become very bored and the roof was hot and I did not want to let down the dignity of my country by going to sleep. I slipped back into the dzongpen's palace and had some more tea.

Tea is, or was, the chief import into Tibet from China. It is pressed into bricks for convenience of carriage on the backs of yaks, ponies, mules, donkeys and men. The consumption of tea in Tibet is enormous, approaching that in British hospitals. It is often used also as coinage.

Now the making of tea is in this wise. You peel a handful of leaves and twigs off a brick, immerse it in a cauldron of cold water and add the soda that is found on the ground here and there in the highlands. The cauldron is then brought to the boil. The mixture is strained and transferred to a churn, where rancid butter and salt are added and thoroughly mixed. Thence it is transferred to a large teapot and consumed in little china cups on silver stands with silver lids. The consistency is that of a thick soup. It is not as unpleasant as it sounds.

The cauldrons, especially in the great monasteries, are enormous. General Bruce, the famous Himalayan wanderer, drinking tea with an abbot, congratulated him on the quality of the brew. The abbot agreed that it was better than usual and sent for the tea-maker to reward him. Unfortunately the official was found drowned in the cauldron, where he had floated undiscovered for several days, buoyed up by his voluminous robes.

Our stay at Shekar was overshadowed by the smallpox epidemic. Smallpox is a very disturbing phenomenon in an unvaccinated and very dirty community. In Shekar there was no true drainage or separate water supply. Washing of the body was unknown, the inhabitants apparently realizing that they were likely to emerge from any bath dirtier than on entry. In such a place smallpox was bound to spread rapidly and to become secondarily infected with every kind of sepsis. The sick and dying lay quietly and uncomplainingly by the path-sides and nothing could be done about it.

These epidemics occurred at intervals of ten years or so, whenever the number of those who had survived the last epidemic grew small by death from other causes and the non-immune population grew thick again upon the ground. The best that I could do was to make several capillary tubes in imitation of vaccine tubes, to instruct some of the lamas and the dzong-pen's clerk in their use, and to send a request to India for supplies of calf lymph. I never heard whether it arrived.

We were most hospitably entertained. In the courtyard, brilliantly painted, a crowd of red-robed novices was drinking tea, poured into dainty porcelain and silver cups from a huge and ornate silver teapot. A lama instructed them as they drank and the abbot sat silently listening. His head-dress of yellow cloth was shaped like the helmet of a Greek soldier. Did Alexander once pass this way? In the temple, brilliant tangkas or sacred banners hung from the ceiling and in the semi-darkness of the inner shrine the face of a gigantic golden Buddha was fitfully illuminated by a ghee lamp carried by a monk whose age was equalled only by his uncleanliness and the odour (not of sanctity) which surrounded him. Round the walls were the images of past abbots, each seated on his own coffin. Thousands of books, dirty and ragged, lined the walls.

Through brilliantly painted corridors and up steep winding stairs we were conducted to the abbey workshop where silver work and thangkas were for sale. For the next hour we haggled over jewellery and teacups and gongs. The scene reminded me of a Moorish market but here there was no mint tea, light and delicious, but the special Tibetan variety.

Above, rose the rock, clothed with steep scree, to the disused and ruinous dzong and farther and steeper still to the still more ruinous watch-tower, a rock climb of moderate difficulty. In the watch-tower the winding stairway was broken and the landings of broken beams allowed sudden downward views of the monastery and camp a thousand feet below. As the sun sank the shadow of the hill stretched out on the plain below with such clarity that we could see our own figures standing on the summit.

We did not wish to stay. We were not afraid of smallpox for ourselves for we were all vaccinated, but the porters were in danger. Getting away, however, was not easy. The mules that were to be our transport animals were due at six-thirty in the morning. Till ten-thirty we sat on packing cases or wandered round the derelict camp. The villagers crowded round, grinning and selling bric-à-brac, occasionally chased away by the cracking of Lewa's whip or a more than ordinarily ferocious charge by our Tibetan mastiff, Policey, who was regrettably given to racialism and had a remarkable power of distinguishing between the local inhabitants and our party. Perhaps it was not so remarkable: the locals smelt differently. The chief muleteer, sighing deeply and doing nothing, wandered about between the few mules that eventually arrived. The dzongpen was sent for but his presence seemed only to add to the prevailing apathy. He wandered about, alone and miserable, from end to end of the camp site, looking as though at any minute he would weep, sometimes finding peace behind a packing case. No one seemed to know what was delaying our departure. Our transport officers circulated rapidly and ineffectually with expressions of extreme efficiency on their faces. Willy McLean went to sleep. Hugh Ruttledge sat on a packing case, wearing his opera hat and looking resigned. Hugo Boustead read the essays of Montaigne. The young Cambridge contingent practised body-line bowling with a mangel wurzel, which I defined as a wanton and indecent attack by one ball on two others. Bill Birnie bought large quantities of jewellery for distribution amongst the beauties of Calcutta. Frank Smythe gave a lecture about what should really be done about it, but didn't do it. Ferdie Crawford had a sudden desire for exercise and disappeared over the horizon. The wireless operators, Smijth-Windham and Thompson, drew a lot of diagrams. I attempted unsuccessfully to sell George Wood-Johnson's washing bowl to the dirtiest of the lamas. Then suddenly, for no obvious reason, we were on the move again.

The way led through very narrow ravines between hills apparently made of brown mud, across a broad river-bed and over a low pass. Beyond the way dipped rapidly to a wide valley and the two ruined forts of Pang-le and the mess tent. It was typical of this very casual and therefore enjoyable journey that we rarely knew from day to day how long our march would be. On this occasion we felt that we had hardly left Shekar. This was lucky because soon snow began to fall and all through the day the transport slowly dribbled in.

We rose early next morning and by five-thirty were on our way. Some wanted an early start hoping for a view of Everest from the high pass of Pang-le. I wanted to leave early because I had come to the conclusion that if I didn't go ahead and choose the next camp site no one else would, or, if someone did, would choose wrongly. The pass, at 17,200 feet, was very cold and there was no view. Eric Shipton and I rode rapidly ahead down a pleasant grassy valley and after about twelve miles had the mess tent pitched in a grove of trees near the village of Tashidzom. There was a little irrigation conduit of clean water and a stork's nest overhead. The trees were bare of leaves, but at least they were trees, rare things in our eyes. The dusty gale had become a gentle dustless zephyr. There were no complaints about the site Eric and I had chosen.

There were plenty of complaints, however, about food. The choice had been left to the secretary in London who had asked us all for suggestions and had taken no notice of them. His motto was 'de gustibus non disputandum'. He had, moreover, turned down a tender from Fortnum and Mason and accepted one from the Army and Navy Stores which seemed to have unloaded on us their most unsaleable goods. We had filled some of the omissions in Kalimpong before starting, but many we found all too late.

We were nearing Everest. A short march took us to Chodzong and next day we entered the Rongbuk Valley. It was a dreary place. On either side grey hills swept down to a deep moraine-filled trough, sprinkled with snow. The sky overhead was grey and a bitterly cold wind blew down the valley at the head of which grey clouds concealed our mountain. We came suddenly upon the Rongbuk Monastery, one of the highest inhabited places in the world. We searched unavailingly for a camping place out of the bitter wind and, failing, erected the mess tent and there took shelter. In the afternoon I walked out and for the first time saw Everest near, stupendous in size, unbelievably beautiful of line and colour. Writers have slighted it and called it a lump. They have lied. Everest was the most beautiful and the most appalling thing I had ever seen.

12 The Everest Adventure

The next day, April 17th 1933, was my thirty-second birthday. We rose later than usual for that day for we were all, sahibs and porters alike, to be blessed by the Abbot of Rongbuk, one of the greatest of Tibetan saints, so holy that he lived chiefly in a glass case. Nevertheless his monastery was decorated with more than the usual number of pictures that would now be described as permissive. They were very beautifully painted but in other ways reminiscent of the Charing Cross and Tottenham Court Roads today.

He was a fat and jovial old man with twinkling eyes who laughed loudly with pleasure at the presents we brought him, a leather attaché case, plastic cups and saucers, some cloth of gold. The porters filed past him, quiet and deeply respectful. Many, including to my surprise our very sophisticated interpreter, Karma Paul, prostrated themselves several times before daring to approach. Each presented a white scarf and a rupee, provided by the expedition. In return each was tapped on the head with a prayer wheel and given a white packet containing some seeds the meaning of which we never knew.

Our turn came. We went one by one to the door of his aquarium, were smilingly tapped on the head, and repeated, whether we were Christians or not, the Buddhist incantation 'Om Mane Padme Hum' – 'Hail Jewel in the Lotus Flower'. We were relieved not to be asked our reasons for wishing to climb Everest; I think they were assumed to be religious.

We pitched our Base Camp five miles up the valley from the monastery at 17,000 feet passing on our way a nunnery and many hermits' cells. The site was on a patch of grass beside a

145

small frozen lake surrounded by moraine heaps. From my tent I could see Everest, white and brown against a blue sky, beyond the scattered remains of the memorials of those who had died on previous attempts. Later the famous yellow band across the upper face turned to gold in the setting sun and left the summit ridge, Mallory's Ridge, blue-black against a sky turning grey with night.

Two days were occupied with the sorting of stores and the testing of the oxygen apparatus that I had designed. It met with much approval because it was light, weighing 12 lb 12 oz, and simple to use. It was except in detail, in fact identical with the apparatus used with such acclaim by the successful expedition twenty years later. Mine was never used.

Our plan was to attempt the ascent without oxygen and, if we failed, try again, this time using it. The monsoon broke during the first attempt, making a second impossible, and my apparatus is still presumably on the North Col or moving slowly down the long glacier to Rongbuk. The evenings were spent in continuous discussion of the plan for the assault, Ruttledge and I tactfully concealing that except for a final question about personnel we had already made our decision.

Wager and I walked up on April 20th to the site of Camp I at 17,800 feet, taking with us a first consignment of stores, a pleasant walk of three and a half hours. I thought we should have made our base camp there, and indeed it later became our advanced base. On the way Ondi, our strongest porter, suddenly collapsed, but was able to return to base. When I returned he was desperately ill. My diagnosis then was pneumonia, but now, forty years later, I realize that he had the mysterious disease of great altitude we call acute pulmonary oedema. I gave him oxygen all night and the next day sent him down with McLean my assistant doctor and Crawford who had a cough and would himself benefit from a spell below in the Kharta Valley.

We had intended to abandon Base Camp on April 22nd but we were awakened early by roars of thunder echoing from the cliffs of Everest, back and forth across the Rongbuk Valley, one peal separated from another by a few minutes filled with the feathery noise of snow falling steadily upon the tents. The camp soon lay deep in snow and though the fall ceased and the sun broke through we postponed our departure. McLean came up from Rongbuk covered with icicles and bonhomie. The Army and Navy stretcher on which Ondi was carried had broken twice on the journey down, nearly precipitating the already half-dead man into the snow: the poles were made of unseasoned deal. But Ondi survived and a few days later appeared at Camp I demanding to join the vanguard of the assault. Twelve young barrhal, ordinarily the shyest of animals, walked solemnly in single file into camp, showing a superb indifference to our presence, clearly well aware that in that sacred valley no life must be taken.

We left Base Camp on St George's Day. Thick white mist obscured the view above us, but no fresh snow had fallen in the night and an occasional brightening of the diffused white light suggested that the sun was trying to break through. The way lay over moraine heaps and across a level stony waste to a long shelf, the old level of the Rongbuk Glacier. We sweated beneath our windproof clothes but a cold wind froze our faces. The first shelf petered out and a climb of fifty feet up steep scree took us to a higher one and to a corner where the East Rongbuk Glacier flowed into the main glacier. We contoured round into the tributary valley and in another half hour reached a broad level area on the true right side of the valley, the site of Camp I. Above, huge red pinnacles rose like Dolomite peaks to 19,000 feet. My tent was at first pitched by my servant in such a way that I had to lie with my head lower than my feet and so near the flaps that snow was certain soon to cover it. After a good lunch of ripe Stilton cheese and dried figs I repitched the tent and felt how good it was to lie there with all my wordly goods within reach of my hand till a flurry of snow undermined my content. The material of the tents was proof against neither wind nor snow. On Kamet the tents, carefully chosen by Frank Smythe, had been made of good material, but not these, and I wondered how we would fare on the upper reaches of the mountains. I decided that if I survived I would buy my tent from the Everest Committee and use it for the purpose for which it had obviously been designed, on a sunny Mediterranean shore. Nevertheless I slept soundly and awoke in a snowdrift at breakfast time.

All next day the stores filtered in from below. In the evening Hugo Boustead and I walked downwards to where, up the main Rongbuk glacier, framed by the flanks of nearer hills, two great snow peaks were joined by a white col as perfectly shaped as the Lötchen Lucke. In the failing light the peaks became a golden pink and great shadows fell across them. The silver and gold turned suddenly to grey and the cold came upon us and we retreated into camp.

Frank Smythe and I set out to explore the route to where, at 19,000, we planned to plant Camp II. We meandered obliquely across the moraine and on to the glacier where we found ourselves in a land designed by a megalomaniac Lalique. Seracs, some of them a hundred feet in height, crowded like fir trees about us, white and green and eau de nil, a chaos of glass. Amongst them Frank and I trudged and climbed, trying to see in this insane forest a glimpse of the way ahead. We cut our way with our ice axes to a moraine that gave some promise of leading somewhere. Here we were overtaken by Eric Shipton, George Wood-Johnson and Tom Brocklebank. We stopped for lunch and discussed the problem of where the Camp II of earlier expeditions lay. After an afternoon of exploration we reached agreement and descended to Camp I.

Hitherto I had gone well, as easily as in the Alps. When we were at about 20,000 feet, my legs began to feel like lead and my balance was poor. I was perturbed by a pain in my chest and my pulse was racing. The sunshine had returned and I lay on a comfortable slab of stone and was relieved to find that my heart slowed and the pain disappeared. I reached camp tired but well, and realized that for the time being I had reached the limit of my acclimatization.

Acclimatization to altitude is a complicated process involving many of the body's organs and physiological processes. Since the Kamet expedition, I had had many long discussions with such eminent physiologists as J. S. Haldane, Douglas and Priestley.

Under their enthusiastic supervision I had spent long hours in a low-pressure chamber at Oxford. Once a careless technician 'crashed' me from a simulated 20,000 feet to earth in a few seconds. I had agonizing earache and was deaf for days. On Everest in 1933 I advised that the average rate of ascent for any climber should not be more than a thousand feet a day. This rule was usually kept, but later I broke it myself with dire consequences.

So next day I rested in Camp I while Hugo Boustead, Eric Shipton, Frank Smythe and George Wood-Johnson followed our route of the day before to the site we had chosen. It was a glorious day, with no wind and not a cloud in the sky. Bill Birnie and I stripped and sunbathed while the porters washed our clothes. Some of them even washed themselves.

On April 27th Hugh Ruttledge, Bill Birnie, Jack Longland and Tom Brocklebank, with myself in the lead, started in great heat and no wind for Camp II. I led slowly and rhythmically. Hearing the perfect rhythm of the party behind me, I was reminded of stroking a boat on the Isis at Oxford. Perhaps there is something akin between rowing and climbing at great altitudes. To the outsider, both are impossible to understand. I went on thinking of Oxford and its problems and when suddenly the north ridge of Everest appeared round a brown hill I found two hours had passed. The way had been greatly improved on our return journey and by the advance party which had gone that way on the intervening day and had embellished it with many cairns. It was no longer necessary to climb, as Frank and I had, a dozen or so of moraines and a selection of glass candle-sticks to find our way. Perhaps because I was no longer tired and now knew where our destination lay, a greater measure of beauty had emerged from the icy chaos. We lunched on Stilton sent by Fortnum and Mason to our 'bijli wallahs', as we called our radio operators, Smijth-Windham and Thompson, at the command of the Indian Army. The local Tibetans who had carried their loads to Camp II came downwards in a bunch, a ragged and cheery crew. They looked on the sahib as a continuous source of merriment and any kind of baksheesh. As ravens and choughs hung around at meal times in the hope of stray crumbs, so did the Tibetans in hope of an empty sardine tin, a piece of silver paper, a biscuit box or an empty lanoline tube, all in a mysterious way to be used again. In the modern world of 'disposables' much could be learned in Tibet. One of them was offered a sardine tin that, to his interest and mystification, actually contained a single sardine. He held it up by its tail, examined it carefully from every angle, smelt it, listened to it as a connoisseur listens to a cigar, took off his goggles and repeated the process, but eat it he would not. When it was explained to him in mime that each of us had many such in our stomachs he laughed appreciatively but incredulously at the joke but still would not eat the monster. The success of the meeting was Hugh Ruttledge, who gravely dispensed an acid drop apiece, repeating to each man the sacred formula 'Om Mane Padme Hum' like a priest at Communion. By each the charm was repeated before he bravely swallowed the offering.

A half hour later we were at the site chosen two days before, lying beside a frozen lake between a moraine and a wall of huge white seracs. It was still intensely hot, with a glare like a furnace. It was strange to hear that the advance party had slept little the previous night at a temperature of $-18°F$. But at four-thirty the sun went down and a great cold came, forcing us into our mess tent where there was soon a comfortable fug of tobacco smoke. Shebbeare told us how in 1924 to discuss future plans was impossible as a quarrel invariably followed. We discussed it all in a most friendly way and a provisional plan was soon agreed.

The stories of the cold on the previous night were alarming. I went to bed at 6 p.m. fully clothed. At six-thirty the porters brought rum and Ovaltine to our tents. I read *South Wind* as a change from *The Decline and Fall* which was my staple reading. The temperature outside dropped to $-15°F$, but I slept soundly. I had an easy day and while Frank Smythe, George Wood-Johnson and Hugo Boustead prospected the route to Camp III, I lay and thought. Lying in bed with the sun shining greenly through my tent, I pondered on the necessity of contrast for the enjoyment of life. I lay on a thin kapok mattress on glacier ice in a sleeping bag that had been inhabited from time to time by various unwashed persons and had itself never been washed in its life of two years. Each night I went to bed physically – never mentally – tired and there is no sensation more delightful. I knew that because I slept with a boulder against my buttocks I would appreciate far more than the constant hedonist the pleasure of the soft mattress I would one day have again. Because I had lived for many months on the tinned food provided by the Army and Navy Stores, occasionally relieved by a delicious bite of the generous 'bijli wallahs' supplies from Fortnum and Mason, I would appreciate all the more the cuisine of Quaglino's, then my favourite restaurant. I would enjoy all the more a quiet stroll through London, with taxis ever available should I grow tired, when I recalled a toilsome trudge across a Himalayan glacier and the knowledge that with no taxi to help me I must reach my tent or die. There a packing case would give me more comfort than the softest sofa. How sad it is that we must travel so gradually between such extremes. I thought as I lay in my tent how delightful it would be if a magic carpet could carry me in seconds from the Rongbuk Glacier to the Hammam in Jermyn Street, where I always ended my Alpine holidays. I would arrive there unwashed and unshaven, still in climbing clothes after a journey in the third class across Europe, often sleeping stretched out in the corridor. My best suit would be awaiting me there. A leisurely Turkish bath, a shave and a haircut, and I would be ready to saunter out into St James's to meet the girl of the moment. Instead I could look forward to the gradualness of the long return across Tibet, the semi-civilization and infinite hospitality of Gangtok, Kalimpong, Darjeeling, Calcutta, Bombay and P. & O. liner before I could issue from the Hammam to find her awaiting me in Ernest Quaglino's cocktail bar.

The route to Camp III lay through the forest of seracs, up a long trough and on to the great open space of the glacier. By May 2nd the advance party was established there. I followed with Hugh Ruttledge, Tom Brocklebank, George Wood-Johnson and forty-seven porters on May 5th under a lowering sky. More snow had fallen and we took it in turn to beat down a track for the porters, often knee-deep in snow until we emerged on to the glacier face, where a strong cold wind blew the snow into our faces, frosted our spectacles and froze our fingers as we donned our crampons. The porters were with difficulty persuaded to go on. George Wood-Johnson led up the glacier with great skill in very poor visibility, but gradually the wind dropped and we found ourselves in Camp III, delightfully situated in full view of the North Col but very exposed to the wind.

It was a bad night. A great wind raged, swaying my tent from side to side, flapping the flies, occasionally penetrating below the floor and after lifting me a few inches, suddenly depositing me again with a bump. The part of the wind's energy not so occupied tore through the tent, chilling my exposed face and depositing on it a fine layer of powdery snow. If I took refuge entirely within my sleeping bag I would be warm and comfortable until the supply of oxygen, already depleted at 21,000 feet, gave out, and I began to puff and seek the air again, to find the wind awaiting me with a fresh supply of snow. The climax came when my tent collapsed altogether and I removed myself and such belongings as were necessary for my comfort to one of the arctic tents. These tents, which had a double shell and looked like Christmas puddings, were the saving of the expedition.

All next day a blizzard blew but in the arctic tents we were warm and comfortable. Further progress was impossible. According to our messman Lakpachedi, who had been with the 1924 expedition, the conditions were far worse than those that sent that gallant band back to base camp. Only a very fit and well-acclimatized party in good tents could sit through such conditions, and we fulfilled these conditions. We decided not to ruin our chances by fighting against impossible odds. We were confident that such weather could not last. One thing only worried us. A contingent of thirty men from Sola Khombu had failed to reach us because of heavy snow on the passes and we feared a serious delay in the establishment of a comfortable camp on the North Col. With a flash of prescience I noted in my diary 'an early monsoon may defeat us'.

Camp III in such weather was too far from the North Col slopes. We felt that a camp at the very foot would give us the chance to work on the next stage in odd moments of better weather. Frank Smythe, Eric Shipton, Jack Longland and I left the comfort of Camp III and taking with us one of the arctic tents made our way along the true left of the glacier until a bulge of mountain forced us out on to its middle, which consisted of a sheet of smooth hard blue ice on which without our crampons we would have been unable even to stand. At 21,800 feet we pitched our tent and sent the porters back. After a good meal we set out in a cold wind and falling snow to explore the route above.

The slopes to the North Col are continuously moving downwards. In the past they had sometimes been easy, but in 1933 they were very difficult. I led, kicking steps in very tiring snow that sometimes took one's weight and sometimes gave way suddenly. Frank Smythe followed on the same rope, carrying wooden pitons and alpine line. Eric Shipton and Jack Longland followed on a separate rope, enlarging our steps and carrying more line. After about twenty minutes the snow hardened and we were able to use our ice axes. After we had climbed about 500 feet the cold forced our return. Looking downwards through the falling snow we could see our tent looking like a huge plum pudding without the sprig of holly. We drove in pitons and roped the route as we descended. Frank and Eric wisely walked down the steps we had made. Jack and I unroped and started to glissade. He reached the foot in safety, but I, travelling over hard snow as fast as I could, ran suddenly into a thin crust, lost my balance, turned a complete cartwheel in mid-air and descended forcibly on my stomach, twisting awkwardly as I fell. I was lucky to escape serious injury and soon rejoined my friends who, helpless with mirth, awaited me below. Next day the weather grew worse. A glance from the tent showed that all our work of the day before had been undone. I was in some pain from my fall and neither Eric Shipton nor Jack Longland was well. Only Frank Smythe, completely fit in every way, chafed at the delay. Bill Birnie, Wyn-Harris and Lawrence Wager came up with another arctic tent, Bill returning with the porters. On the next day I too descended to Camp III, not because of my accident but because Hugh Ruttledge needed my professional advice about the party.

The party now was distributed thus:

Base Camp The bijli-wallahs, Smijth-Windham and Tommy Thompson.

Camp I   Empty.

Camp II   Shebbeare with a sore throat, poorly acclimatized.
           Crawford, better in health and aching for the heights.
           Brocklebank, working hard on stores but poorly acclimatized.
           McLean as exuberant as ever.
           Wood-Johnson, very fit.

Camp III   Ruttledge with a bad sore throat and rather ill.
           Birnie, very fit.
           Myself, now recovered from my accident and very fit.

Camp IIIA Boustead, poorly acclimatized.
           Longland with a severe cough but otherwise well.
           Shipton with laryngitis but otherwise very fit.
           Wyn-Harris, Wager and Smythe, all in the pink of condition.

I awoke at Camp III and through the window of my tent saw the North Col bathed in light golden sunshine against a dark blue cloudless sky. The temperature was −18°F. The day remained sunny and we hoped that a day of uninterrupted sunshine might make it possible for the party at IIIA to do some useful work on the North Col slopes. But a message came down from Smythe that the snow was too dangerous for any advance.

May 12th was another brilliant day, the night before enlivened by the sight of the full moon over Everest. I had completely recovered from my muscular strains but there was no way in which I could help and I lounged through the day stripped to the waist. Birnie paid a social call at Camp III and came back with the glad news that Smythe, Shipton, Wyn-Harris, Wager and Longland had made the North Col. We had another fine day. The transport arrangements were reorganized, Crawford taking over at Camp II and Birnie above. I don't remember that any decision about this was taken by our leader or by the soviet we had become. Birnie tacitly assumed responsibility and nobody argued. Shebbeare, our official transport officer, the most lovable, imperturbable and knowledgeable of men, but in his fiftieth year, had shot his bolt and never came above Camp II again, though he resisted McLean's order to descend to Camp I. We missed him sorely.

On the next day the roping of the North Col slopes was completed on yet another sunny day. I sent Hugh Ruttledge down. From my point of view, life was made easier by the fact that he, the leader, never questioned any medical decision I might make. On May 14th the weather began to turn against us and the wind was hellish but Shipton, Smythe, Birnie and Boustead got away from Camp IIIA and established Camp IV on the North Col and I joined them at IIIA. Two pieces of news filtered up from below. The first breath of the monsoon was reported from Ceylon and counselled speed. But forty-six porters had come from Sola Khombu and had marched straight through from Rongbuk to Camp II. That night a blizzard such as none of us had ever known began to blow. Our arctic tent, hitherto a model of stability, swayed and crashed. Outside the wind squealed and wailed and the snow hissed horizontally past. When light came I could see the sun outside shining not on the white snow but on a surface of hard grey ice across which raced a fine white cloud of blown spume. After a morning of indecision the advance party, Smythe, Shipton, Birnie, Wyn-Harris and Boustead decided to brave the wind and went up to Camp IV to stay. Longland and I descended in twenty minutes to Camp III to find it windless and bathed in sunshine. We had had little to eat above. The assistant sirdar Sonum Topge (not officially a cook) produced for us a memorable meal of ham and eggs. The bijli wallahs had sent up a Stilton cheese at exactly the right stage of ripeness. We lay in the sun and found it difficult to leave for the wind and cold of Camp IIIA but at last we tore ourselves away. As soon as we left the moraine for the open glacier the wind met us again and blew gustily through the evening and the night, and continued in the morning.

Once more I set foot on the North Col slopes, the gale doing its best to blow me from my tracks. Despite the blowing snow the route was clear, festooned now with ropes and even, in the steepest place, with a rope ladder. At this point Smythe had shown his superb icemanship. The ice wall here was forty feet high, the lowest ten feet overhanging, the upper thirty almost vertical. Up this Smythe had cut steps supported at first by an ice axe firmly planted against his buttocks. It was the only climbable spot along a two-mile length of ice cliff. But for this chance and Smythe's brilliance we must have returned defeated. It took my party two hours to reach the foot of the ladder he had planted. Wager and Longland ascended it while I sat below roping up the porters one by one. Wager found the steps above the ladder destroyed, so for an hour or more I stood on two small steps on a very steep snow slope in deep shadow, growing colder as a continuous shower of ice chips descended on me from above. But at last the job was done. My feet were completely anaesthetized and I left the others and made for Camp IIIA, where Crawford and Brocklebank had arrived. I had no after-effects. Optimism prevailed, but the gale still blew.

During the night the noise of the wind gradually lessened and gave place to the sound of gently falling autumn leaves. All next day the snow fell and to ascend to Camp IV was impossible. We lay in the comfortable arctic tent like pips in a gigantic cantaloupe. In the evening the hurricane returned. Once or twice in the night I woke to find the tent swaying ominously. At two o'clock there was a resounding crash and the side of the tent fell in. Longland, who had very virtuously insisted on sleeping in his own leaky Meade tent to leave more room for the rest of us, slept on undisturbed. The remaining four of us sat up and looked at one another with a wild surmise. We knew that if we could not erect the tent again it was the end of us. In such cold and in such a gale survival would have been impossible. With no word spoken, Wager and I climbed out into the night. It was fairly light but bitterly cold. The moon and stars were partially obscured by light clouds scudding violently across a dark blue sky. The mountains stood around vaguely self-illuminated. The wind was so strong that we could hardly stand. Knee-high for me, shoulder-high for the shorter Wager, a thick layer of driven snow raced horizontally, so that only his head was visible, apparently decapitated. All the guys of the tent had given way, but after an hour they were replaced and the tent was secure though lop-sided. After this unpleasing interruption I slept uninterruptedly till seven o'clock.

But the gale did not sleep. On May 18th it continued furiously and although we knew that food must be getting short at Camp IV, to get porters up to the North Col was manifestly impossible. With gigantic labour we straightened our lop-sided tent and sat and hoped for a lull. On May 20th it came. I led to the foot of the ladder where I remained for an hour and a half roping up the porters two at a time. The last three were of the recently recruited Sola Khombu men. They refused.

Up to this point they had both pleased us and amazed us. Unacclimatized, they had carried loads on their first day from Rongbuk to Camp II and after a day's rest had continued to Camp III, some to Camp IIIA. But the rope ladder was too much for them. Had our own original men refused, my quaint mixture of English, Urdu and Khaskura might have been adequate, but the men of Sola Khombu spoke only Sherpa, a dialect of Tibet. One laid down his load and retreated down the hillside, leaving me with the uncomfortable task of supporting it on the unstable snow. The others would go neither up nor down. Much time was spent in polyglot and useless abuse. Longland let down a rope and with great labour pulled up the abandoned load. The remaining two at last responded and decided to attempt the ascent of the ladder. Number one climbed it so unskilfully that he swung it sideways and his load slipped from his shoulders. Going to his assistance, standing with two toes on a slippery rung and my left hand round the upright, I suddenly received the whole weight of porter and load on my right arm. Extricating myself from this difficult position involved considerable effort at that altitude but eventually he reached easier ground above. The second man did better and I followed him up the ladder to arrive exhausted at Camp IV.

Camp IV lay in a bergschrund, filled with snow, below a huge overhanging cliff of blue ice. It was a somewhat squalid place. While I was on the ladder a party had attempted to establish Camp V, but had turned back too soon. Controversy raged, but to resurrect it forty years later would serve no useful purpose. Hugh Ruttledge struggled up on May 21st and decided that on the following day I should join the advance party (although I knew I was insufficiently acclimatized) and with Wyn-Harris, Boustead and Birnie should attempt to push the site of Camp V to the agreed altitude of 25,000 feet. I had not had the chance of following my own rule of acclimatization, but in the difficult circumstances could not refuse. The plan now was that after establishing Camp V and Camp VI, Wyn-Harris and I should reconnoitre Mallory's Ridge and, if possible, go for the summit. We were not expected to succeed, for by that time opinion had swung definitely in favour of Norton's Traverse as the best line of ascent. Eight porters only were to remain at Camp V for one night and continue next day to Camp VI, to be brought down at once to Camp IV by Birnie and Boustead. Meanwhile, Frank Smythe and Eric Shipton who were not only very fit but outstandingly the best climbers of us all, were to move up to Camp VI in support of Wyn-Harris and myself. Longland and Wager were to be in support at Camp V. Wyn-Harris and I having climbed the mountain or (as seemed more probable) failed, would return, report to Smythe and Shipton at Camp VI and descend to Camp V, whence Longland and Wager would have descended to Camp IV. Smythe and Shipton would then climb the mountain by Norton's traverse.

A very steep snow slope led to the top of the North Col. Above this the north ridge of Everest is of scree, easy to walk on, edged on the right by a wide stretch of snow. A rocky precipice fell away to the left. Wyn-Harris led with Wager, Longland and myself behind him and Boustead in the rear as beater-in for the porters. They were going splendidly but for one who was suffering severely from stomach-ache: I asked Longland to take him back to camp. At about 24,500 feet I began to feel my lack of acclimatization. I found it difficult to keep up with Wager who was going strongly and averaging 600 feet an hour. We did fifty-minute spells of climbing, then resting for ten. I longed for those rests as never hart for cooling streams. I took two breaths to each step and each step needed all my will. We came across George Finch's camp site of 1922. There were four oxygen cylinders lying there, their white paint still bright and the valves still shining, so dry is the air at these altitudes. I took a swig of oxygen. The first effect was a sudden increase in the light. I saw more sharply and colours became brighter. Around lay the tent, collapsed but still bright green. The wooden pegs were still white and the brass untarnished. A few empty food tins lay there, their labels still clean and legible after eleven years. I pocketed a Kodak film, but alas it was unexposed. I dismissed a thought that had been in my mind that I should retreat, and for a few minutes I climbed with alpine ease. But the effects did not last. Soon again I was forcing every step. The porters too were beginning to lag and take frequent rests. It was largely the necessity to keep them moving in the icy wind that kept me moving too. Tsinerbu, an old Kanchenjunga tiger, as proud as Lucifer of his past record, suddenly decided to go no farther. I pretended not to recognize him and lifted his goggles. 'What,' I said, 'Tsinerbu! Oh, Tsinerbu!' 'Atcha, Sahib,' he said, and on he went again.

At one o'clock, at about 25,700 feet by aneroid, we came upon an obvious camping place. The rest of the party was in good order. Wager immediately set about levelling the ground. When the porters arrived they began to build a wall as neat as any builder's. I was utterly exhausted. My pulse was irregular and when I felt for my heartbeat I found it two inches out of place. The burden of my thought was heavy. I had been given the chance of making the first assault on the summit of Everest which looked very close, but I knew that I had shot my bolt. I stripped off my spare sweaters, handed them over to Wager, and with a very real lump in my throat demoted myself to the menial post of escort to the porters returning to Camp IV. I wasn't a good escort. Within minutes they were well ahead, romping cheerfully down the mountainside, and I was alone.

The going was easy to a trained mountaineer, scrambling over rocks about as easy as the Grib Goch ridge on Snowdon, interspersed with patches of snow. But I was a sick man. In every patch of snow I fell over and rested a while. At last in a very comfortable spot, sheltered from the howling wind, I decided that I had had enough. I was warm and comfortable and the view was superb. If I stayed where I was I would fall comfortably asleep. I had no wife or children for whom I could feel responsible: my parents had five other children and, though I knew they would mourn, they would lose only a small proportion of their offspring. I decided to stay.

I am reminded of what sometimes happens in a hot bath on a winter morning at home. One lies there comfortably and there is no hurry to get out. Then suddenly one is out of the bath with no conscious effort to leave it. I do not remember any such effort, but suddenly I was struggling downwards again, falling again in every patch of snow, but rising at once when breath returned. Then below me were the tents of Camp IV bright green against the snow.

To get out of Camp IV we had cut our way with our axes almost horizontally along an almost vertical wall of ice. To maintain our stance along this wall, with the ice above us a foot or so away on our right and that below dipping at the same steep angle to unmeasurable depths, needed exquisite balance. It had presented no great difficulty in the freshness of the morning. Now my sense of balance had deserted me. I could not stand upright on a horizontal floor of snow. Yet I remember walking with complete confidence along the steps we had cut and no foot wrongly placed; then my memory fades. I had reached Camp IV.

So, while others battled for the summit, I rested at Camp IV near the North Col. The snow continued and on May 23rd a series of small avalanches fell on our tents from the upper lip of the bergshrund below which we lay. Ferdie Crawford, who in 1922 had had the unpleasant experience of descending the North Col slopes in an avalanche in which seven porters had died, expressed extreme disapproval of our position. Brocklebank brought up the telephone that connected us now with Base Camp, where the bijli wallahs were now in touch with Darjeeling. The first news was that George Wood-Johnson had descended with bad tummy trouble to Base Camp. There followed a series of weather reports which were for the most part unhelpful. Though the persistent bad weather, worse we gathered than any previous expedition had experienced, was said to be due only to temporary Western disturbances, one thing emerged – the monsoon was upon us.

May 24th was a day of uncertainty and discussion. The snow continued at Camp IV and a wind of great ferocity raged at Camp V. Through our telescope we could see that no advance was being made to Camp VI. But on the next day the sun shone. Wyn-Harris and Wager left Camp IV with six porters to replenish food at Camp V, hoping that Birnie and Boustead and their porters would be descending. We were disappointed. During the morning the whole of the upper part of the mountain became untenable by reason of thick snow and a howling gale.

During the night of May 26th two small avalanches fell on our tents. This had several times happened in previous days without much comment, but night terrors prevailed and were supplemented by the cold (horribly cold) light of day. It seemed likely that the coming of the monsoon would rapidly make the slopes below impossibly dangerous. It was decided to move Camp IV to the top of the North Col, where it would be safe from avalanches and to evacuate to Base Camp all those who were not actively engaged in the assault. The plan was sound. No former expedition had experienced the embarrassment of having eleven members at the North Col, all but one well-acclimatized and with gigantic appetites. The supply position was difficult.

It was decided that Frank Smythe (in command) should stay at the North Col with Eric Shipton, Wyn-Harris, Lawrence Wager, Jack Longland and Bill Birnie, the rest of us retreating to Camp III. I was very ill. Happily the snow was in unexpectedly good condition. Below the rope ladder I began to feel better, presumably because of the increasing amount of oxygen in the air. The blue ice cliffs and velvety slopes of snow, now turning steely grey in the failing light, made me realize again how lovely was the world about me.

At Camp III, at only 22,000 feet, I slept like a log and awoke at seven o'clock on a still and sunny day. Willy McLean said my heart was still dilated, but I didn't mind. By helping to establish Camp V 3,000 feet above Camp IV and 500 feet higher than ever before, I felt I had done my job. I planned to lie in the sun for a day and then to descend leisurely to Base Camp, doing on the way what small odd jobs I could and there to laze a while and attend to the wants of the casualties coming from above. I hoped that in a few days I would hear that the mountain had been climbed. If it had not I was determined to return myself to the attack. An acute dilatation of the heart can recover very rapidly.

So I left Camp III with Hugo Boustead. It was a funereal descent, for his toes were slightly frostbitten and, remembering my descent from Kamet, I sympathized. It was a day of blue skies and white cumulus clouds, very still though at over 20,000 feet. We dropped down the glacier, easy going to the trough. Where with great labour I had cut steps in ice for the porters so short a time before, the snow lay thinly on the scree. Little streams flowed here and there, appearing suddenly out of the snow and disappearing again beneath it. The seracs were smaller now but even more fantastic. They seemed to have moved a little away from one another as though each feared the collapse of its neighbours. Between them had appeared little paths and inviting winding stairways. Occasional small lakes had replaced white tracts of snow. The wrecks of two huge seracs showed that the fears of their neighbours were just and that soon the route would be very dangerous.

Out of the trough, the way that I had helped to stamp in the grief of my heart and the sweat of my brow was beaten hard and firm by the passage of many laden porters. When we reached Camp II we found it lying on moraine, not on ice and snow as when we saw it last.

Lachman Singh, whom we had left in charge there, was ready for us. Our tent had been scrupulously cleaned. Wooden boxes had been arranged like a table and chairs, and tea was on the hob. On a side 'table' he had arranged some old illustrated magazines, a tin of tobacco, and a box of matches. Jeeves himself could not have done better.

We tarried for half an hour and started for Camp I. It had been a tedious task for Frank Smythe and me to find the way up the complicated glacier from I to II. Now there was neither ice nor snow. Boustead and I walked as on a gravel path and as we went began to experience the subjective effects of having more oxygen to breathe. As on the descent from Kamet, colours became brighter. The air seemed to be thicker and felt glossy in the throat. Faint aromatic smells came to our noses and we heard again the sound of running water. A comfortable contentment, a relief at turning once more towards the valleys where life could flourish, dispelled the disappointment we both felt at leaving our friends on Everest, still unclimbed.

It was almost dark when I stumbled into Camp I. I was a half hour ahead of Boustead and had time to have a good meal ready, pea-soup that did not taste of peas, sardines, galantine of chicken, dried figs and a Stilton cheese I had looted at Camp II, all washed down with rum, a meal fit, we thought, for a king. The Whymper tents, open to the night air, seemed enormous after our cramped space in one-fifth of an arctic tent, and it was good to sleep alone.

On May 29th, unable to break ourselves of the habit of waking early to discuss the weather, we were away by 8.30 a.m. It was well for me that I had the frost-bitten Boustead with me to limit my speed, for the pain in my chest returned for a while, but was forgotten in the utter content of returning at last to a reasonable altitude. When we reached the end of the side glacier where it entered the main Rongbuk Glacier we looked back at the final pyramid of Everest. It appeared at first to be bathed in sunshine and still peace. One small fleecy cloud moved in a leisurely way along the summit ridge. I timed it: it took fifty seconds to travel a measured mile.

Downwards, the snow peaks that had stood along the valley had become brown and yellow downs, purple in the cloud shadows, flecked with the pale green of moss cushions and young juniper. Far ahead the hills were of so bright a purple that one thought that heather grew at the valley's end. A bird sang. Two tortoise-shell butterflies found the first flower, a large white gentian. A spider darted from under my foot. Life had come again.

But not peace. At Base Camp, now loud with the calling of pigeons, I found Tommy Thompson, busy with his radio, and George Wood-Johnson sick with a gastric ulcer. Neither seemed to have observed that into the camp had crawled not only the invalids amongst our porters, who were very few, but those who had just had enough. In every nook and cranny they hid nervously, sharing our provisions with a multitude of Tibetans, male and female, who were often to be seen descending the valley carrying mysterious loads. To the indignation of Karma Paul, who had probably been drawing a substantial income from these illegal practices, I held a parade of everybody in camp, expelled the local spongers, separated from the mob those porters who had served us well at the high camps and ordered the others to Camp III with what delicacies I could find.

The order was not to their liking. They stood in a long line of protest, but it was clear that only one trouble-maker was active. Without him the others were unlikely to sacrifice the high pay they could expect. I called him out of the throng and ordered him to be first up the trail. He refused and I felled him with one blow on the jaw. A roar of laughter came from his former supporters, who picked up their loads and left, still laughing. Their happy laughter could still be heard long afterwards as they neared Camp I.

I settled down to the first good meal I had had for six weeks, but afterwards there was still much to be done. The ponies were obviously starving. Boustead needed help with his arrangements for departure. Wood-Johnson had to be put to bed and given medicine. I gave a long broadcast to Hugh Ruttledge at Camp III. We had a great farewell dinner to Hugo Boustead.

At last I remembered that I was an invalid with a dilated heart and went thankfully to bed.

After the joy of a night without awakening, untroubled by the foetid unwashed proximity of my companions and their loud panting breaths, I was awakened by the first rays of the sun upon my tent. The air that blew between the flaps excited and enlivened me and no longer sent me deeper into my sleeping bag. Whatever might be happening on the mountain above I had two or three weeks of warmth and good food and real air in which I could laze or zoologize before facing again the discomforts I only then fully realized now that I had left them.

I talked to Camp III on the radio but I learned nothing. Camp IV was apparently incommunicado, and nothing was known about doings above. I took off my clothes for the first time in six weeks and had my first bath. I was horrified by my wasted muscles and the thick sprinkling of spots on my white body and thighs, the result of excessive sweating. In the afternoon news came through at last. On the day before, Wyn-Harris, Wager and Longland had established Camp VI at 27,400 feet and Longland had brought the porters safely down through an intimidating blizzard. On this day, Wyn-Harris and Wager were last seen making good progress at 7.00 a.m., but after that cloud had obscured the view.

As we learned later, they had examined the ridge route (Mallory's Ridge), and in particular the second step. They said it was like the bows of a battleship and at that altitude unclimbable. So they continued along Norton's Traverse, below the ridge, and again made good progress with little snow on the rocks. But they had spent much time on the ridge and knew that they had no time to reach the summit. At 28,100 feet, with the end in full view and very near, they were forced to turn, dropping down again to Camp VI, where Smythe and Shipton were already installed, and down to the North Col.

It was on this day that Wyn-Harris and Wager found the famous ice axe, lying on a sloping rock an hour above Camp VI. It must have belonged either to Mallory or Irvine, who had disappeared hereabouts in 1924. No mountaineer in such a place would have willingly abandoned his axe. What had happened was the subject of long discussion for many weeks, but we were finally agreed that the spot where the ice axe was found must have been the scene of an accident. Here the slabs of rock are steep and are sloped the wrong way, like tiles on a roof; there are no belays round which a climber can twist the rope for the safety of himself and his companion. If climbers are roped together in such a place, the fall of one means the fall of both. Mallory and Irvine were probably roped, though we cannot be certain. They were certainly roped when Odell saw them earlier. We can then picture the scene. Mallory, the brilliant expert, would have been leading. He hears Irvine, the tyro, slip behind him, lays down his axe, takes the rope over his shoulder, holds it with both hands and takes the strain. But the slip continues and the two fall together into the almost bottomless depths.

But did the fall occur on the way up or down? We shall never know with certainty but I have little doubt that it was on the way up. We know that they were making for the ridge route that Mallory always favoured, which came to be called by his name. I accept the verdict of Wyn–Harris and Wager that the second step on the ridge is unclimbable. In 1924 the pair may have abandoned this route and continued below the ridge on the slowly rising traverse called after Norton who always favoured it. If they had reached the top by Norton's Traverse they would not have descended along the route on which the axe was found, but by a more direct route lower down.

We shall never know definitely what happened to Mallory and Irvine, but such evidence as there is suggests strongly that they died on the way to the summit.

May 31st was one of the longest days of my life. The mountain was invisible. Thompson and I spent our time between the wireless tent and the mess, calling Camp III every few hours, but always hearing 'V.A., V.A., V.A. – no message for you yet, Base Camp'. George lay in his tent in great pain from his gastric ulcer which my primitive medicines did little to relieve. We tried to read and tried to write, kept from the bottle only by the still living hope that we might need the brandy for celebration. In the late afternoon seven of the eight 'tigers' trotted down the moraine into camp, all fit and well but ignorant of events above. I gave them food from the sahibs' rations and sahibs' tents to sleep in. Thompson and I settled down in the 'bijli tent' and sat in a maze of wires and little black handles waiting for the message that we felt must come at last. Our poised pencils were shaking and I said, 'If they have got up, I think I am going to cry.' Thompson said, 'Me too.' We heard only a multitude of irrelevant sounds – mosquitoes buzzing, loud whistling, the roar of a lion, faint faraway strains of music, a brain-fever bird in distress – and then suddenly the high bird-like chirrup that was Camp III. 'A message to Base Camp. Owing to heavy clouds and snowfall today no news has been received of climbing parties. No cause for anxiety'.

June 1st came. It was 'V.A., V.A., V.A.' all the sunny day. We built a bathing pool to occupy our time. June 2nd was the same and the suspense became almost intolerable. At last, in the late afternoon, we were in touch again. 'Wyn-Harris and Wager descended from North Col to Camp III yesterday, going well. Slopes still safe despite monsoon current. No news yet of Smythe and Shipton. Their tent can be seen from Camp IV. Strong wind from N.W. over summit will prevent movement today.'

In fact, Smythe and Shipton were confined to their tent for a day but made their attempt on June 1st. Conditions had radically changed. The monsoon had deposited thick powder snow upon the mountain. At that altitude snow does not bind beneath one's boots but slides off down the mountainside. The going was terrible. After a while Shipton was forced to turn, but Smythe went on in steadily worsening conditions. At about the point reached by Wyn-Harris and Wager in fair conditions two days before he retreated, with the summit only a thousand feet away, but the day far advanced.

On the morning of June 3rd, Ruttledge came through again. 'Phone from Camp IV late yesterday stated Smythe and Shipton returned safely from Camp V . . . Camp IV being temporarily evacuated. Conference at Camp III today. Next plan depends partly on medical advice, partly on weather. Now definitely proved upper part of Everest very difficult. These first two defeats due solely to climbing difficulties. We are not yet beaten.'

I telegraphed to Ruttledge advising a period of recuperation at Base Camp. On June 4th Smijth-Windham trotted down the big moraine from Camp III, looking very fit. He had left Camp III before the conference but had no doubt that Ruttledge intended to take my advice and order a general retreat. I bathed in our new swimming pool at a temperature of 35°F.

These, I noted in my diary, had been lovely days at Base Camp. All day the sun shone from a blue sky piled high with cumulus clouds. I turned my face from the mountain with a total absence of the bitter disappointment I had known at Camp IV and feasted them on the purple hills at the valley's end. A great quiet lay upon the camp. The privacy of one's spacious Whymper tent was a treasured luxury. I had come to like my friends more and more and the greater the discomfort and mental strain the more I came to respect them. But even such companions can be too close in body if not in mind. Here one was free from the appalling sordidness of life at great altitudes, where five or six men must share a tent large enough for three. In the arctic tent at Camp IV the floor was covered always by a horrid mélange of sleeping bags, boots, dirty underclothes, paper, dirty plates, knives, forks and spilt food, the whole stuck together by ancient lumps of Kendal fruit cake or overturned tins of condensed milk. In this mess one lived and ate and slept. It was a lovely thing to have one's own clean and tidy tent, to have one's meals sitting on a chair before a table spread with a bright tablecloth. One forgot the recurrent frightfulness of food cooked by oneself on a Primus stove that seldom worked without long coaxing. Here there was no need for economy of fuel and when thick ice prevented the morning plunge, a hot bath would always be produced.

The peace was soon to be disturbed. Day by day, the party descended in various stages of dilapidation and my services were in continuous demand by day and sometimes night. A rather elderly porter named Kipa who was convinced that he had died at Camp VI and was brought back to life by a sharp kick on the behind followed me about the camp, in his eyes the adoration of one who has been restored to life by an effective if somewhat indelicate miracle.

By June 10th the weather was definitely characteristic of the monsoon. Everest became white. But there was a general feeling that we had not yet shot our bolt. Smythe, Shipton, Wyn-Harris and Longland of the high climbers were fit again. By keeping McLean in bed and escaping examination I declared myself fit, for I felt that in another attempt a doctor must be with the party and McLean was not well enough to go. Ruttledge, Brocklebank and Crawford had not been high and were in good order. Of the original fourteen, eight were therefore willing to have another try at what I was beginning to realize was a hopeless venture.

The plan was for Crawford and Brocklebank to set off ahead and re-establish the camps. Two days later Shipton, Longland, Ruttledge and I were to go to Camp III and wait there till Camp IV was in being again. Thence Shipton and Longland would advance. A day later, Smythe and Wyn-Harris, now the fittest couple, were to 'go through'.

It was time we left. Vegetables were running low. An assignment from Kalimpong had been looted on the way. Llakpa, an attractive little lady who had travelled with us from Phari to where her route branched off to Sola Khombu, had several times appeared with a load of eggs and onions, but she was too small to keep us well supplied. Moreover, we knew that sometimes a fine period will suddenly occur during the monsoon. If this lasted long enough, wind and sublimation could clear the snow from the mountain. If we were near enough when this happened, another try could be possible. At the moment, the upper part of the mountain was obviously impossible.

On June 13th Ruttledge, Longland, Shipton and I started again for the upper snows. The weather was fine but for an occasional flurry of sleet. Ruttledge, despite his age, and Shipton, fit as a fiddle, went ahead at a good pace; Longland, with 'tummy trouble' and I, unduly breathless, at a slower pace. I found it convenient to stop frequently to collect specimens of the little cushion flowers that were beginning to appear and of the spiders that were my particular care. I had frequent attacks of breath-lessness, not especially associated with steep stretches of the way but often on level ground. The old feeling of constriction in the left of my chest began to return, and I knew what this meant, but I arrived eventually at Camp I, where I ate and slept well. Next day the weather showed signs of improvement. Ruttledge and Shipton raced ahead but once more Longland and I fol-lowed at a more sober pace. We reached Camp II in three hours to find that the lake had doubled in size and that the tents now lay not on snow as when we had seen them first but on smooth rock. We made Camp III on the next day in brilliant sunshine and our hopes rose. I took the lead and led, unduly slowly for the tigerish Ruttledge and Shipton, through the serac forest. The seracs were much smaller and had lost their old magnificence. Till we reached the smooth surface of the glacier I went well though slowly, but I then began to wonder whether graduated exercise was really the best treatment for a dilated heart. The heart thought not and I resigned the lead and fell well behind the other three. Arrived at Camp III I was relieved to know that I had done all that was expected of me. But I slept damnably, afflicted by that unpleasant disorder of breathing known to physiologists as Cheyne–Stokes respiration

On June 16th Everest was still, despite the fine weather we hoped would clear it, an even white. Wyn-Harris and Smythe arrived very fit from below but Crawford and Brocklebank came from above. They had gone two-thirds of the way up the North Col slopes. The whole area was deep in new snow and beneath it the old snow had degenerated into powder. An avalanche had obliterated most of the ladder. The col was unclimbable.

A conference of war took place on June 17th. The choice be-fore us seemed to be: (a) to go home now; (b) that a small party should remain at Camp III in the hope of a change in the weather; (c) that we should retire to Base Camp and wait and see; (d) that we should retire to the comfortable Kharta Valley for a month; (e) every possible combination of (a) to (d). I took the view that from now on there was no chance of the upper mountain and the North Col being possible at the same time again this year. The whole mountain was coated in fresh powder snow which made the col too dangerous and the upper part of the mountain too difficult. The appalling winds that we had experienced in the first assault would probably, in the monsoon season, not recur and would therefore not sweep the mountain clear of snow. In the damp air of the monsoon, the sublimation that could earlier turn the white mountain into a red one, would not take place. By the time the mountain was clear again the winter would be upon us. To stay at Base Camp to observe the weather for future expeditions was, I said, a waste of time, for no monsoon was like another. As to the Kharta suggestion, I could see no useful object. The party would probably recuperate there faster than at Base Camp, but with a few exceptions it was fit and down there it would be impossible to observe conditions on the mountain or to seize the opportunity for a further attack.

We left and on June 22nd descended towards Base Camp. More flowers were out. All round Camp I, where when we saw it first it appeared impossible that life could exist, were growing small blue delphiniums smelling strongly of musk and a little mauve primula that was new to me. Between Camps I and Base Camp there grew saussurea, a small mossy vetch, a dwarf yellow ranunculus and tiny white cushion flowers with pink centres. Base Camp was less pleasant than before. Sunny days were few and there was no morning brightness to tempt me into the bathing pool, into which apart from me no one but Longland had ever ventured, the rest treating the exercise with derision. Each day at one o'clock the whole sky became black and there fell an unpleasant mixture of rain and snow. On one day there was a violent thunderstorm, great peals of thunder, synchronous with the lightning, echoing from side to side of the Rongbuk Valley and re-echoing from the cliffs of Everest. June 26th was Longland's birthday and we broached the case of champagne we had brought to celebrate our victory. The first bottle, owing to the low pressure, exploded with such violence that its contents probably landed at Camp VI. More cautiously thereafter we opened each bottle pointing downwards into our canvas bath, helping ourselves by dipping our glasses therein. For many months we had tasted no alcohol. Perhaps too at 17,000 feet, heads may be weaker. Soon a concert began which for some curious reason assumed an entirely religious character. Everybody was supremely happy, but through all the noise, with tin mugs, basins, champagne corks and every possible missile flying about their heads, the bijli wallahs Thompson and Smijth-Windham continued heroically to decipher a long coded message. They read it and the party became suddenly sober. Williamson, the Political Officer in Sikkim, told us that there was very little chance of permission from the Tibetan Government for another expedition in the following year and advised us to stay on. The reactions of the different members of the party were interesting to observe.

A telegram was sent to the Everest Committee suggesting that Ruttledge, Smythe, Shipton, Brocklebank, Crawford and myself should stay on in the hope of an improvement in the weather. Had I felt the faintest hope of this I would willingly have stayed indefinitely with such companions, for between us six there had never been a trace of disagreement. I enjoyed the lazy tent life and my health was rapidly improving. But it was not to be. A telegram arrived ordering us home.

While the camps above were being evacuated under the orders of Shebbeare, I became very lazy. My diary would remain for days unwritten. My collecting bottle became a scene of congestion where moths, beetles, flies and spiders lay jostled together in death. Each morning at seven-thirty, Lewa, who, though Chief Sirdar, had decided with his usual inexhaustible desire to work to appoint himself my personal servant in lieu of Ang Tensing, who was up the glacier with Shebbeare, would tie back the flaps and allow a flood of sunshine to inundate my tent. I would lie lazily watching the moraine above on which a tame hermit lived and above which could be seen, when not obscured by cloud, the tip of Everest. After a while Ruttledge would appear in my rhomboid field of vision and disappear behind my heap o medical crates. Then Lewa would reappear and, hissing like a groom, would lay out my razor, sponge and soap. With nothing in my prospective day to cause me worry or annoyance, no work, no conflicts, but only a uniform spectacle of lazy sunshine, I would ease myself out of my bag and dive into the cold but no longer freezing pool, shave and don the shirt, shorts and shoes that were my only clothes till evening fell. After breakfast I would lie sunbathing at a discreet distance from the camp and its attendant vivandières, lazily smoking and persuading such small creatures as immodestly approached my naked form to find a last resting place in an empty matchbox. So the day would pass, quietly but without boredom.

Meanwhile the camps above were gradually evacuated and on July 2nd we were ready to depart. By noon the transport animals were assembled. There followed the usual delay inseparable from eastern travel. Every load was the centre of furious argument. Occasionally the whole crowd of yak herds stood apart and held a protest meeting. The Tibetan as an individual is full of charm except when looting liquor, but in the mass he develops a skill in obstruction incredible to one who has never travelled in central Asia. By four o'clock however we were away, leaving only ten men wrapt in windy argument on the difficult question of dividing the last three loads between fifty-four yaks.

We took a last look at Everest and walked towards the purple hills.

13 Retreat from Everest

We camped that night, July 3rd, near the Rongbuk Monastery and the next day set out on the fourteen-mile march to Chodzong. The Rongbuk Valley, which on the way up had seemed the dreariest on earth, had greatly changed. Instead of a biting wind and flurries of snow there was a light warm rain, laying at last the intolerable Tibetan dust. The desert had begun to blossom in small bright tufts between the stones, islands of sedum, purple vetch and pale blue iris. The hills along the valley, on our upward way black and dismal, were brown and yellow and in the distance brightest purple. Chodzong had had little grass when we passed that way before. Now the valley floor was brightest emerald interspersed with yellow buttercups, pink primulas and scented violets.

The invalid contingent had not arrived from the base hospital at Tashidzom to which I had sent them. I wanted badly to see the Kharta Valley but instead Ruttledge and I set out to examine the situation, leaving the others to go over the Doya La to Kharta. After about two miles we came to what had been a trickle on our upward journey but was now a raging torrent that we crossed with difficulty. Below the ford the valley became very fertile and we rode through fields of flowering mustard towards pale brown hills over which snow peaks showed pale blue beneath lowering clouds. The rain fell steadily.

About five miles from Tashidzom we were met by the local squire, riding a gorgeously caparisoned mule and proudly wearing the green Homburg hat that we had given him on our upward journey. At first (for speech between us was impossible) we thought that this was an example of the great courtesy we had

174

learned to expect from Tibetan gentlemen. But no; hearing on the local grapevine that our party was bound for Kharta, he was hoping to catch us at Chodzong to extract payment for grain supplied to our ponies while we were 'up the hill'. The history of these ponies, quartered at Tashidzom while we were in the high camps, had been a sad one. Knowing from previous experience that the oriental thinks no shame to add to his income at the expense of a horse's stomach, my first act when I went down to Base Camp had been to summon all the ponies from Tashidzom for examination. They were skeletons, and on making inquiries I found that the ration ordered for them was about half of what I thought necessary. I doubled the ration and sent them down again. Thereafter they not only resorted to short rations again but amply lined the pockets of Nerbu, our chief seis, a revolting old man whose dishonesty was equalled only by his inefficiency. Birnie, arriving at Tashidzom three weeks before, had taken all in hand, but the condition of the ponies was still very poor and Smijth-Windham's was so weak that it could carry him no more.

About a mile from Tashidzom we were met by Birnie in a delightful grove of willows, as peaceful a camping ground as we could hope to find. Violets grew thickly in the grass and scented the whole scene. Most of the invalids had largely recovered and were, I decided, fit to take the road to Gangtok. I wanted to stay a while in the warm green world, but I had to get them away. We left the route of our upward journey and followed the main valley of the Dzakar Chu, which flows east and south towards the end of the Kharta Valley where it flows into the Phung Chu. We moved slowly, for McLean was feeling very weak and our guide did not know the way. Five miles from Tashidzom we had to call a halt at a large farm. The farmer and his family, including three pretty daughters who had never before seen a white man, came out and regarded us with huge amusement. One of the daughters particularly took my fancy. Taller and slimmer than most Tibetan girls, she had a more Aryan face, a tip-tilted nose and a lovely figure. One small firm grimy breast occasionally peeped through the folds of her still dirtier robe. She showed

175

in her amusement at our quaint appearance a row of perfect teeth unusual in Tibet. Later I told Karma Paul about her and he immediately offered to go back and fetch her for me. 'But, Paul, supposing she would come, what would happen on my return to England?' 'Sahib, it is simple. You give her a few rupees and her travelling expenses home.' 'But she would never then be able to marry in her own village.' 'You are wrong, Sahib. She would have great honour.' However, we left it at that.

My invalids were doing well except Wood-Johnson and Mc-Lean. Wood-Johnson's gastric ulcer was not healing and McLean was too ill to be of any assistance to me. We continued our pleasant way and on July 9th rejoined the main party at the end of the Kharta Valley.

Natural laziness, medical responsibility, a feeling that nothing now mattered much, combined to end my diary. I am left only with vignettes of memory.

Of the day when Jack Longland and I, stark naked, raced our ponies across a great green plain and, forgetting our state, into a village of which the inhabitants had never seen a white man, least of all a nude one.

Of the night when George Wood-Johnson's gastric ulcer threatened to perforate and I spent the night beside him with the immediate prospect of acting, in Willy McLean's state of incapacity, as anaesthetist and surgeon both.

Of the border between Tibet and India where the wind was bitter and strong and with our packing cases we built a long wall to protect the tents. The natives came in the night and stole the top layer of cases, which included almost all my zoological specimens, all except the few still in my rucksack collected on the previous day. Karma Paul and I went to the nearest village, paraded the villagers, and told them that if the boxes were not found their children would die of smallpox. They wailed and fell on their knees, screaming for mercy. The boxes were not found. I do not know whether they got smallpox.

Of our arrival at the beginning of the road to Gangtok where I knew that the responsibility would drop from my shoulders

and I put my heels into my horse's flanks and galloped into town
to the kind and competent Dr Henriques who immediately sent
out an ambulance. We dined that night with the King and his
charming Tibetan Queen.

Of a weekend with Sir Malcolm Hailey, the Governor of the
United Provinces and his delightfully unconventional Italian
wife. Rumour said that he had been offered the Governorship on
condition that she was sent home; that he refused; and that he
got the job just the same. One day when I was having a morning
cocktail in the A.D.C.'s room she entered in a girl guide's uniform and a state of high dudgeon. 'I,' she cried, 'have troubled
myself to get all the badges I can, shooting, first aid, everything,
even good conduct. And now they say that officers must not
wear badges. Ha, but see, I fox them.' She lifted her skirt, and
there they were, neatly sewn on to her bloomers.

Of the day when I called on my cousin Roland Raymond, a
medical officer in the Royal Air Force. I found I was billed to
play hockey for the Army against the R.A.F. Never having
played hockey I was released, but with difficulty. I remember a
hectic drive to the playing field on the pillion of Roland's
powerful motor-cycle, but not much else till a mob of somewhat
mimsy officers took me to the station and attempted to install me
in the private compartment of the Military Secretary. Foiled in
this effort they decided to debag the General, but I dissuaded
them from this and attempted entry into another compartment.
They then lifted me into a horizontal position, held me there till
the train began to move, and propelled me head-first through
the happily open window, landing me, still horizontal, on the
lap of the astonished inhabitants. This I gathered afterwards,
was the traditional farewell of the Royal Air Force in India reserved for its more distinguished guests.

Of lunch with the Viceroy, the Marquess of Willingdon and
his fury at the Everest Flight. This journalistic effort had as its
moving spirits Colonels Blacker and Etherton, a couple of most
entertaining adventurers, who, when the latter was British
Consul-General in Turkestan, had succeeded, according to
Lord Willingdon, in selling to the Standard Oil Company the

non-existent oil rights in Turkestan, which were of course not theirs to sell.

Of the night in Bombay that I always think of as a whiff of chrysanthemum. The Japanese House, easily recognized by the lantern that hung in the cherry tree at the gate and flood-lit the clean white walls, was quiet and peaceful after the filth and horror of Grant Road. The old lady who owned it, gnarled and twisted like a bonsai, was voluble and lucid in a wild mixture of languages, Urdu, Japanese, English and a smattering of anything convenient. She showed us into a large room two-thirds of the floor of which were covered by an immense divan, on which after, of course, removing our shoes, we gratefully reclined while three charming girls in national dress, all comely but one of exceptional beauty, with the fragile loveliness of the geisha of dreams, knelt at our feet and kept our glasses filled with Bass. Occasionally, assured that our immense thirst was temporarily allayed, they would slip off the divan on to the floor and divert us with little tinkling songs sung in their little tinkling voices.

> *Tora chini, tora char,*
> *Velly fine gentlemen yes you are!*
> *Queen Victoria rule de lan'.*
> *Queen Victoria velly fine man.*

At last they were allowed by the old lady, who kept a most careful eye on what went on, to sit beside us. Emboldened by Bass I put my arm round the waist of the most beautiful of the trio. She stiffened but made no effort to escape. I talked to her soothingly in English, of which she didn't understand a word, and she gradually relaxed and lay close within the crook of my left arm with one hand in mine, and occasionally even took a sip from my glass. Sleep overcame me.

When I awoke Keiko was still there, very close and fast asleep. I kissed her very gently on the forehead and she half awoke and snuggled still more closely. I cannot remember how long we lay there, but suddenly I realized that we were alone and that dawn was creeping into the room. I kissed Keiko again and she fully awoke, gave me one embarrassed glance and fled. I slid down the divan, put on my shoes and made for the door. The others were all under the cherry tree. I was horrified to realize that Bonham, who was a little drunk and whose conversation in fluent Urdu was sometimes difficult to follow, was attempting to buy Keiko, not for himself but for me. 'My friend,' I heard him say, 'is extremely rich. A little matter of a few thousand rupees is nothing to him. Surely just for a night that would be a good profit.' The old lady, far from being shocked, was rocking with laughter, refusing every offer. Frank departed to some unknown destination. The old lady pushed Bonham with unerring instinct into a house across the road in which he wished to make what we would now call bioavailability studies, from which he did not emerge for many hours. Me she detained. Drawing me into the kitchen she attacked with admirable directness.

'Do you love Keiko? She is sixteen but she is still a virgin.'

'Madam, I can recognize innocence when I see it,' and (pompously), 'I can respect it.'

'But do you love my little granddaughter?'

'I think she is a charming girl.'

'I would like her to marry you. She can sing and play and cook and will make a good wife. Also she loves you and so do I. You would make her happy.'

'Honourable grandmother, I am honoured and very touched. Never has so much honour been done me. But it is impossible.'

'Why?'

'Because I leave for England in a few days.'

'She can be ready to go with you.'

'But she will not be happy in England. She doesn't know the language; she will be lonely without friends; the climate is cold and damp.'

'As to the first, she will soon learn; she will not be lonely with you there; our climate is too hot and either too dry or too wet.'

'Nevertheless, after so short a friendship I cannot agree, tempting though your proposal is.'

179

Moments of Being

'When will you be back again?'
'Perhaps next year.'
'I shall keep her for you.'
'No, you must not do that. I cannot be sure that I can return.'
'I know that you will return.'
But I never returned.